MORE LOVE TO GIVE

with love &
best wishes

Helen x

MORE LOVE TO GIVE

A story of Secondary Infertility,
IVF and the desperate quest for another child.

HELEN DAVIES

© Helen Davies, 2017

Published by Town Bridge Press

www.secondaryinfertilitymatters.com

A CIP catalogue record for this book is available from the British Library.

ISBN 978-0-9955794-0-8

Book layout and cover design by Clare Brayshaw

Prepared and printed by:

York Publishing Services Ltd
64 Hallfield Road
Layerthorpe
York YO31 7ZQ

Tel: 01904 431213

Website: www.yps-publishing.co.uk

Dedication

To my beloved family, Jason, Zac, Xavi and Anya.

Zac, may you one day read this and understand that it was our overwhelming pride and love for you that made us want more like you. You were always enough. You are the light of our lives.

Anya and Xavi, may you one day read this and understand just how much Daddy and I loved you before we even knew you. You are both precious gifts that we will forever look upon in awe and with pride.

Jason, my husband, my best friend, my rock and companion through all of this. We did it. "Impossible, but true."

About the author

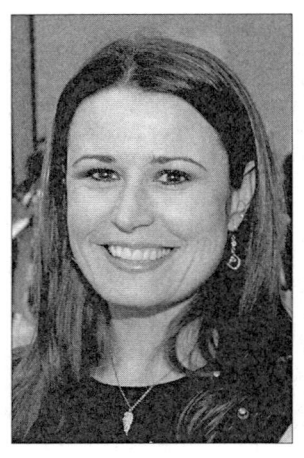

Helen Davies was born in Croston, Lancashire, a village still close to her heart. She studied Public Relations in Leeds and a career in PR and Marketing followed in Liverpool, Manchester and Hull. Helen has been a PR Manager, a Marketing Communications Director, partner in a Property Development firm and run her own PR and Marketing agency.

Helen is passionate about supporting couples and raising the profile of the term Secondary Infertility and all its complexities. She runs support website **www.secondaryinfertilitymatters.com** manages a blog and social media pages of the same name, writes for Fertility Road magazine, supports Hull IVF unit as Patient Representative and works closely with Fertility Network UK as Media Volunteer on the subject. She also speaks to medical students and drug companies to give an insight into what fertility treatment is like from a patient's perspective, and is a regular contributor in the media.

She now lives in East Yorkshire with her husband Jason and children Zac, Xavi and Anya. She founded the online gift store The Lovely Keepsake Company following the birth of the twins in 2013.

Foreword by Susan Seenan, Chief Executive, Fertility Network UK

"I'm delighted to have been asked to write the foreword for 'More Love to Give'. Secondary Infertility is very common, and yet we don't talk about it nearly enough and I hope this book will not only help to raise the profile of Secondary Infertility, but also help people to understand the impact.

Secondary Infertility can be every bit as painful and difficult to deal with as Primary Infertility and couples suffering from Secondary Infertility deserve support and understanding, just as much as anyone who is trying to conceive for the first time. Just because you have a child doesn't mean you can switch off the longing to have another baby, but there is often a sense of guilt about this – a feeling that you should simply be grateful for the child you have when others are still trying for a first.

Often, there can be the added pressure of existing children asking why they can't have a brother or a sister. This can exacerbate the emotional impact felt when trying for a second baby: not only is there the pain and longing for another child, there is the feeling of guilt that you can't provide a brother or sister and that your only child may be missing out. In addition, for couples who have conceived naturally first time around it may be incredibly difficult to deal with the fact that it's not happening for them in the same way again.

I hope anyone reading 'More Love to Give' finds comfort and reassurance in Helen's words, in particular that they should not feel guilty for wanting another child. I also hope that anyone in this position who isn't successful in having another child can move forward and positively embrace having an only child; it took a long time for me to accept that we were only going to have one child, but there are positives when you can invest all your time and energy into your one and only child."

Introduction – I'd really love a pudding

"Just because I've just enjoyed a main course doesn't mean I don't want, shouldn't have or don't need a second course. I'm full after my meal but I'd still really love a pudding."

It was an analogy I played over and over in my head every time I heard my friends say: "Well at least you have Zac" or "Just remember how lucky you are to already have one baby". Time and again I wanted to scream back at them: "Haven't you ever felt full after a big dinner but still been desperate for a pudding?" It was the only way I could think that I could ever make them start to understand how I was feeling. But I didn't say it, ever.

I was well into my fertility treatment when I decided to write down my thoughts, feelings and experiences. I didn't find any support in books or forums that offered comfort for a mummy who wanted another baby. The IVF community seemed to focus on couples trying for a first child, which only sought to ram home to me my feelings at that time, of guilt, greed and shame at wanting another. I didn't want another Mummy to feel as I had.

It wasn't until I completed this book that I found there was actually a term for how I felt and for our predicament. The fact that I had been so isolated because I was unaware of the name 'Secondary Infertility', because nobody dare speak about it, only reinforced my desire to talk to more people who might also be battling through gruelling fertility treatment whilst trying to bring up a family. I didn't want that family to feel alone.

When friends see that you have now started your family it seems weaning is the time for a prompt to pry into when you're going to pop the next one out and when your child starts school, it would seem this is an 'acceptable' trigger to start questioning why you have failed to provide a sibling as yet. People can be cruel in their assumptions and interrogations sometimes. I wanted to share how it feels to be on the receiving end.

Secondary Infertility, as I now know it is known, is extremely common with some reports suggesting it perhaps counts for a third of the one in six infertility cases in the UK, and it's on the increase. We may never know the true extent of the number of couples affected by Secondary Infertility. Why? Well fertility clinics don't record or share figures, the lack of funding available second time round mean many couples won't even visit a fertility clinic in the first place, and lastly but perhaps most importantly, many couples don't realise they have a problem that may need intervention, they simply believe they are just struggling. The real figures are potentially huge.

The emotions, practical hurdles and everyday situations that test you as you try for a second child are different to those when you try for your first. And yet, unlike with the first, you can't escape reminders of babies when you have a toddler round your ankles all day, or a nursery room your child has grown out off that is gathering dust waiting for its next resident.

It's definitely true that most people think that if you can have one child you can have another. Why not? It's probably this reason that there is often a lack of empathy. If you have a child, you are quite rightly looked upon as having been lucky and so in forums or support groups where you might seek support when you are trying for your second, there is often an unwelcome stigma. In fact, you're just not welcome. How dare a Mummy complain about wanting another child when she is lucky to have one already?

I recently read: "why is it that when a couple decides to add a second child to their family everyone is happy for them and thinks it's great? Nobody questions whether or not their first child was enough, and nobody suggests they shouldn't try for another because they are lucky! But when a couple needs treatment to help them conceive another child, all of a sudden it becomes a big deal. It's an issue to want more and they are overwhelmed with suggestions to "just be thankful for the one you have" and "maybe you aren't meant to have another", or their friends assume it's selfish to pay for treatment when their child has needs so they are told "focus on the one you have".

It is such a double standard. They are really hurtful statements but they are dished out all too frequently. Just because someone needs treatment to make the family they dreamed of before infertility become a reality, doesn't mean they deserve it any less, don't believe they are fortunate already or aren't unbelievably thankful for the beautiful child or children they already have.

It's a lonely place; almost a 'No Mans Land'. You feel so isolated and distant from the fertile, baby world that you long to be part of and yet you are cast aside from the infertile community, who shun you as they seek just a little of what you are already have. Nobody in any broad fertility forum or chat room wants to hear the pain from someone struggling for a second, you simply aren't welcome to share your thoughts and feelings.

I know, and always did know, that we were blessed with our first child Zac. I'm not sure I would ever use the word 'lucky' as we tried for three years and had 10 months of fertility drugs before we finally conceived. In 2007, our stars collided, our angels were watching over us and after both medical and non-conventional treatment, my body finally responded giving us our much wanted and loved baby.

Not once, did I ever, think or feel that Zac was not enough. Nor did I ever feel ungrateful or complacent that we had our son. He filled my life in so many ways but I did feel our family wasn't finished and I did want him to have a sibling. I wanted another child for him as much as for myself. They were simply feelings I could not turn off.

Five years later, as our ride on the gruelling IVF rollercoaster, without success, began to take its toll, I started to believe that the more love I felt I had to give should indeed be directed at Zac, rather than potential future children. It was becoming more and more apparent that the treatment was distracting me from the attention he obviously needed. Those are days I can never get back and that feeling is something that will always weigh heavy in my heart.

I did start to think that Zac would be our only child and finally, after three years trying and 14 months of intensive treatment, that thought and the blessing that was Zac in our lives, slowly and quietly began to feel enough. The longing did start to subside. If we were to be a family of three, finally, after everything we had been through, I could start to feel that I might find it within me to feel content. We had been through so much, I didn't feel I could put myself or family and friends through any more and so fortunately as that realisation started to sink in the thought of doing more to have another child was, for the first time, starting to be a real turn off instead of a dream. It wasn't what I wanted and I knew I would have setbacks and the real yearning would never go away, yet the four rounds of IVF in 13 months made me reconsider my life, what I had and how I could potentially be permanently damaging it all whilst chasing another dream. It started to feel like too big a risk to take.

I have known the pain of seeing friends and family members have babies, sometimes two, during the time I was trying for my first child. I know that when you are in that situation, having just one child would make you feel like you had received the earth. And it did, for a while. I haven't written my story without remembering those days but I wanted to try to shed some light on a similar painful set of circumstances and emotions that are sadly too often ignored or underestimated. Wanting a brother or sister for your child and feeling that you are failing has its own demons. And for anyone standing in judgement of my story, perhaps who are themselves desperate for a first child, I would say that their predicament is just one of many reasons Secondary Infertility hits couples hard. I knew your pain, I knew I was blessed already when others weren't, but I couldn't help how I felt.

Perhaps a better analogy after all might be a bar of chocolate instead of a pudding. I love chocolate. When I have a bar of chocolate I feel excited and lucky to have it, I savour each mouthful, enjoy every chunk but as soon as it's all gone, I want another. As much as I enjoyed eating the whole bar, I love it so much I could always scoff another!

I truly loved and enjoyed what I had, but it only left me wanting more and for that I should not feel guilty. It is the perfect analogy to describe my desire for children.

A seat round our table, a place in my heart, I simply always felt I had more love to give.

Our star was born

"We've done it! Jason, we've done it!"

It was all I could think to say, the only words I could find and the emotion at just hearing myself say them was almost overwhelming.

I was lying in a crucifix position, with nurses holding me down at both sides, as my body shook violently, caused by the adrenalin racing through me. I had no other words. I was just solely focussed on what had just happened that, despite nine months warning, had still taken me by complete surprise. There was nothing else that came into my head other than utter amazement at our triumphant achievement. We'd done it!

We had prayed for this, hoped for this and imagined what it would be like for so long. It was something that happened to other people, something that everyone around us had done, some more than once and now, we had finally made it too. The last four years suddenly shrank into one insignificant, easily forgettable chapter of our lives, the disappointment erased and it was this moment now that would be the one we would remember forever.

Jason, who had been at the other side of the theatre, was now stood next to my head as I remained laid out on the table. I wanted to jump up and put myself in his arms so he could wrap them both round me and we could hug for the longest time. We were in a room crowded with people, yet only the two of us knew just how huge an achievement this was.

"It's a boy!"

A boy! A beautiful, baby boy.

I longed to feel our new baby's warmth in my arms and yet I decided not to hold him on the way back up to the ward. I was worried the nurse might frown at me for not volunteering to hold him, but after a 12-hour labour and then an emergency C section, I still felt weak and exhausted. After all this time, there was no way I was going to risk anything happening to my baby. Especially with Jason in charge of the wheelchair!

Back in our own room on the labour ward, his tiny face peered out from the Perspex cradle next to my bed. Perfect. The enormity (and there is no greater word I can find in the thesaurus to express this) of the feeling that I had produced this tiny person kept rushing through me with an intensity I had never felt before. This was different. This was much more. This was "wow". This little baby, this person, this new life was produced by me, my body and I promised him there and then that I would cherish him forever.

For months after, I found myself repeating the same words to people: "I can't believe how powerful the feeling that I have for him is." I knew motherhood was supposed to be an amazing experience and it was something I'd dreamt of for many years but if I'm honest, I really think I underestimated just how overwhelming the love you have for the child you produce is. To say you'd walk on hot coals for them is an absolute understatement and I'm sure I'm not the only mother to think that.

Yet for me, I do think there was a far more poignant element to it.

I did it. Me. I managed to produce a child. There were times when I really thought it would never happen. We had been trying for four years. What was wrong with me? It was me after all, not Jason, that had the fertility problem and the thought that I was letting him and my family down was almost unbearable. Yet most of all, not being able to fulfil my own deep longing for a child that had built up in recent years, was absolutely heart-breaking. It had developed into a pain, a real anguish and as the months passed by, that pain deepened.

Torture is far too strong a word, but I had felt tortured. It seemed everywhere I looked there were babies or pregnant tummies. Friends, passers by, even TV soap characters, it seemed everyone around me was embarking on the baby chapter of their lives, except me.

And yet, at that time, I had become adept at being able to see other people's existence as completely separate to mine and to compartmentalise my feelings so that for most of the time, when I heard about friends' pregnancies or when I'd see bellies full of arms and legs whilst out shopping, most of the time, I managed not to get too upset. Knowing how much I was hurting at that time, how could I not feel happy at the joy they were obviously feeling? I wouldn't have wished my frustrations on anyone else. Of course I wished it was me and there was always a pang of regret but amazingly, I never used phrases like "it's not fair". They had their lives and I had mine. It was my life; my problem and nothing that did or didn't happen to them would change my situation. I had to feel happy for them, and largely I did.

At times though, the longing, the waiting and the sheer bloody frustration would simply overwhelm me. Anything could set me off, and most of the time it was just triggered by my mercurial hormones.

If I had just had a period or done yet another negative pregnancy test, there would be days, sometimes weeks later when any mention or reminder of someone else being pregnant would send me into a foul mood with unstoppable, silent tears.

I remember one night when it all got too much. One of my friends had hired a box at Sheffield Arena to watch Justin Timberlake and all the girls were really excited. We had our own bar, own food and private viewing area. It was a fantastic night out and I was thoroughly enjoying myself singing and dancing with everyone. Towards the end of the concert one of my friends pulled me close and whispered: "I've not told any of the others yet but I'm pregnant!" I was thrilled for her, gave her a huge hug and promised not to breathe a word. I squeezed her hand and smiled down at the gorgeous Justin as I thought about her good fortune and the brilliant, beaming smile on her face. I was genuinely delighted.

I then stood looking at all my girlfriends dancing in the box around me. There was eleven of them and each one was a Mummy. They had all known the joy of telling people they were pregnant, carrying a child within them and yes, the pain of childbirth I guess! But every single one of them had a child; everyone except me.

In silence and now standing still at the back of the group with a self-poured quadruple Bacardi and Coke in my hand, I watched and listened to Justin belting out his final tracks and I sobbed. Nobody saw and nobody knew but my heart was breaking and tears were streaming down my fully made up face. I had another drink and then joked with some of the girls as they saw me pour yet another. Why couldn't I be a Mum? What the hell was wrong with me?

We had been trying for three years without success. I'd been taking fertility drugs for more than a year now and hadn't had a drink for ages, so this blow out was a rare occasion. It was also ill advised. What I didn't know that night was that I was actually three weeks pregnant!

It was a fairly uneventful pregnancy, no real complications, a couple of causes for concern but nothing serious and nothing that would have put me off doing it all again.

That's perhaps a strange statement to make given that I vomited on average six or seven times a day for the entire nine months. I'd drive with sick bowls on the passenger seat and throw up as I'd drove. I had to run out of client meetings or run from my desk to the ladies with just a moments' notice! And yet, I loved having my baby inside me and couldn't wait to meet it. "Pip", as we affectionately called 'it', was the centre of my world before he or she even arrived.

Pip was due in the middle of January and as I got bigger towards Christmas I tried to slow down, wind things up at work and focus on preparing for our last Christmas as a couple. It was bizarre because it seemed in every shop I went into, all the 'baby's first Christmas' gifts were jumping out at me. They seemed to be everywhere willing me to buy them. It was obviously exciting but I had to focus on this Christmas and just the two of us, there would be plenty of time for those gifts next year.

Pip had other ideas. It was the night before Christmas Eve when my waters broke! It was hard to believe it really was my waters and as the contractions started to get stronger later that morning, the nurse had to stress to us both that we had better get used to the idea that we were going to have our baby that day. And so, three weeks early, gate crashing Christmas 2007, Pip arrived!

As we stared back at him now in his Perspex cradle, we could hardly believe we finally had our baby. We also realised we hadn't decided on his name and that we'd now started to call the baby, not the bump, Pip. There was no way I was going to let that nickname stick for my beautiful baby boy.

Zac Gordon Davies was welcomed into the world on 24 December 2007.

For some reason that year, loads of our friends and family were away from home, either on holiday or spending Christmas with their families in other parts of the country. With Zac being early and his birth happening so quickly in the end, nobody except immediate family knew that we were even in hospital. Jason's phone calls and texts to our friends that Christmas were magical and their delight and excitement was infectious. I will never forget so many people saying how it was the best Christmas present and how they'd toasted our baby's health around dinner tables all over the world. Despite spending Christmas Day in hospital it really was a very special and memorable Christmas.

Zac

Every parent is biased but my Zac is one of the most wonderful children I have ever met. He has a beautiful compliment of gentle sincerity and a caring, loving nature mixed with a comical, impish sense of humour and infectious energy that is pure joy to be around. I can honestly say he has made me laugh for one reason or another every day of his life.

I wouldn't be true to this book if I didn't talk about the first nine weeks of his life honestly though. He wouldn't settle, didn't sleep, constantly cried, in fact he screamed so much he gave himself a hernia and popped his belly button out! I was dead on my feet, struggling to feed him with no sleep and on one occasion, devoured 8 packets of Hobnobs and 36 chocolate mini rolls in just 48 hours! I blamed it on a desperate need for energy!

A neighbour introduced me to a phrase she said she knew I was searching for: "bone tired". She wasn't wrong! As soon as she said it, I knew exactly what that expression felt like and realised it gave me the words to perfectly sum up how I felt to my midwife, who wisely advised me to stop breastfeeding and get him on formula. He soon settled, still never slept well, but at least Jason and I could now start to feel a bit more human and start to build our new life with our new addition.

Zac instantly became our main focus. We carried on doing what we wanted to do and were determined not to lose our identities and to some degree we achieved this. We always took him to what we called 'grown up restaurants' not play barns, we took him to the shops we wanted to visit and we still tried to spend time visiting our friends. Inevitably though, we had to consider his needs more and more and as he grew we'd find ourselves visiting places to entertain or stimulate him in those early years. Places we'd never had the excuse of visiting as a young couple but were now actually really enjoying.

Farms were the best and standing at the many five bar gates near our house pointing at sheep, cows and horses was actually really interesting. Who knew? I became an avid tractor spotter and would often get excited and shout out that I'd could see one, only to realise I was alone in the car!

You don't really realise your baby is growing, changing or becoming a toddler, then a child. You notice each milestone in isolation. You're constantly willing them to develop, learn new skills and enjoy new experiences. They get teeth, start to walk, start to talk and after doing all that, only then, at nearly two years old, did Zac start to grow hair!

I was putting more and more clothes that he'd grown out of away in boxes and we found ourselves constantly going out and buying new shoes or new coats. He'd use a new word, expression or gesture that we'd never heard or seen before, the kitchen door was filling up with artwork he'd produced at nursery and then he started forming his own new friendships with children we'd not introduced him too.

He had his own little world, he was developing so fast and it was only when I stopped what I was doing one day and watched him chatting away to his toy firemen, that I realised my baby really had grown up. He was a little boy now. We found ourselves encouraging him to the next milestone each day and before we knew it, we were looking back and he had raced through them. The little baby we once knew wasn't around any more.

Of course it goes without saying that I still loved him, that he was still the centre of my world, in fact, the more I got to know him probably the more I adored him. I'd often say to him he'd always be Mummy's baby, but it saddened me and only reinforced just how fast he was changing when he'd retort most sternly "No Mummy, I'm not a baby, I'm a big boy!"

A new chapter was dawning

When Zac was five months old I started a new business, getting back into marketing consultancy that I'd done some years before. In some ways it was exciting but in many ways it was one of the most stressful periods of my life.

I could write a whole chapter about why and how I ended up starting this business with a new baby just a few months old, but in summary, I needed to work, it was what I was good at and with no close family living nearby, I felt I had no option but to work for myself as I needed the flexibility in case Zac was ever poorly.

Zac had been booked into the Old School House Nursery in the next village since I was five months pregnant. I'd always imagined I'd go back to work and reserved him a place as soon as I could, as I knew of its excellent reputation and extensive waiting list. I wanted the best for my baby and I immediately felt excited as soon as I went for my preview visit. I was already excited at the fun my 'Pip' would eventually have there.

It would be fun for Zac for sure, but for me, my apprehension at how much it might hurt to take my baby to nursery actually only just scratched the surface to what it actually felt like when the time came. I will never forget the gut wrenching pain, real physical hurt inside at having to leave him and force myself to walk away, down the path back to the car, knowing I wouldn't see him for 9 whole hours.

Would he understand what was happening? Would he wonder why I was leaving him? He was mine, I was all he knew and I knew him so well. There was only me that had spent so much time with him so how would they know when he needed a nap, when he needed his bottle or most worryingly, that he wasn't actually being smothered when he pulled his cuddly elephant, Little Blue, over his face, but rather it was how he liked to fall asleep!

I knew I sounded frantic when I first left him, in fact actually I have to confess, the first morning was just too unbearable and Jason had to take him! But thereafter, I could hear in my voice that I sounded almost unhinged and hysterical leaving the girls with advice and instructions on how to care for him. They never let it show if indeed they thought the same however, and I realised as I quickly began to know and trust them, that they were more than used to mummies like me and were well used to desperate ramblings on the baby room doorstep!

Both Zac and I soon settled in quickly to the Old School House Nursery routine and felt that the girls were almost part of our extended family. They gave us advice on teething, chicken pox symptoms, weaning and much, much more and I can honestly say I don't know where I'd have been without those girls. Leaving your child is difficult at the best of times but to feel unsure about the people you're entrusting your baby to must be horrendous. I never, ever felt this way and in fact I loved those girls so much for the love they so obviously felt and showered on my baby. Despite the initial, understandable nerves and apprehension, I realised that Zac's life was being enriched by his nursery experience and he was surrounded by people who genuinely cared for him.

My business was growing by now. I'd merged my consultancy with a friend's business and together we'd re-launched, taken on staff and the client base was growing quickly. Nobody booked in meetings for me before 9.30am as I didn't want to have to drop Zac off at 7.30am only to sit in city centre traffic for an hour just to get there for 9am, especially when I couldn't collect him till 6pm. So I dropped him off later, missed the traffic and got to the office just after 9am. That was my life now, new priorities.

We all settled into a routine at work and at home. Jason and I managed juggling drop off and pick up and we even seemed to cope with looking after Zac when he was off sick, which seemed to be every other day as soon as he started nursery! We also, miraculously, seemed to cope with getting up for work in a morning despite having been up four or five times in the night putting dummies back in, changing wet sheets or mopping up vomit (or worse!).

Being a mum was working out pretty well. I remember my Mum saying, "You're a good Mum, and you're coping well, better than I thought you would."

Strangely, ignoring that she obviously thought I was going to be rubbish, I was thrilled that she said this. After all, she'd had 33 years experience and I thought she'd done a pretty good job herself!

Work got busier, Zac moved from the caterpillars to the butterflies and then to the bumblebees group at nursery and family life was working out better than we could ever have imagined.

I'm not sure when I started to think about another child. I do remember a time when I was clearly thinking Zac was still too young, that I wanted to devote more time to him and that it was too early to leave the business yet. But as for when all those feelings reversed into then wanting another baby, I'm not quite sure. However, we had never taken contraceptives. It had taken nearly four years to conceive Zac so there was no way I was stopping Mother Nature if she was on a roll, that was for sure.

I guess the yearning for another baby must have been gradual; perhaps it almost crept up on me. Zac's friends began talking about baby brothers and sisters and one by one, all bar one, all of his friends had a sibling. Zac would often talk about them, or in fact other babies in the baby room. He'd ask, "what's a brother?" or "have I got a baby sister?" and then, as his vocabulary grew, so did the inquisition!

I think perhaps it was an accumulation of factors that planted the seed and changed my mind without me realising. Zac growing out of clothes, casting aside more and more baby toys, in fact in general, it was probably his growing into a little person in front of me, becoming independent and not really needing me as much.

In some ways I guess his growing up left a space for a baby but it also created what felt like a hole in the family. We'd never planned the size of our family in terms of numbers and yet suddenly it felt like there was space for someone else and as Zac grew, I guess he kind of made space for another baby to come along. And so, the die was cast, the decision made and the real yearning for our second child began.

The fun is in the trying

It had taken nearly four years to finally have Zac and we had been trying for two and a half years before I was finally diagnosed with polycystic ovaries. After two trials of different fertility drugs, the second being Clomid, we successfully, naturally conceived which was a tremendous feeling. In simple terms, one of the symptoms of polycystic ovaries is the difficulty in creating and releasing eggs, something the drugs stimulate you to do. Having being diagnosed I didn't want to waste any time now, presuming that I'd still need the same stimulation.

After a few months of trying without help, it seemed silly to continue for any great length of time knowing of my previous difficulties. By this time, I was 35 and whilst I still felt young, in fertility terms I was no spring chicken.

I was excited to be starting trying again. It seems strange to think I felt like that, given all the heartache and length of time it had taken us to conceive Zac, but it is true to say that when I consciously acknowledged that we'd actually made the decision to try for another baby, the thought of having another was definitely thrilling. I'm sure Mother Nature was playing her tricks and wiping my mind of all the negative aspects of having a baby and letting me look back on those months through rose tinted glasses, just as she does to many women after a difficult birth, but I was definitely excited at the thought that very soon we would have another little person in our house.

Having been treated privately before, we had no problem calling the fertility clinic again and getting an appointment with our consultant Professor Killick who was based at the Hull IVF Clinic. Again the thought of seeing him was nothing short of exciting. There are some people in this world who are very, very special and I'm sure anyone who has been through fertility treatment successfully, will have someone they hold dear in their heart, someone who was their saviour, their hero. Professor Killick is mine.

When we did our positive pregnancy test with Zac and after reality sank in as the shock subsided, all I wanted to do was see, hug and kiss Professor Killick! 6 weeks pregnant and just 2 weeks after I'd done my test, I did just that! Back into the waiting room of the clinic, waiting to see him, it was all I could do to hold back the sobs, trying to get my head round the fact that I was sat in that room again, as I had dozens of times before, but now I was pregnant! By the time the Prof appeared at the door, I could hold back the tears no more and flung my arms round him in grateful appreciation.

The occasion was made all the more special that day, when he asked if we'd like a "cheeky peek" at the baby. Warning us that a scan so early may in fact show that the pregnancy was potentially not viable, with our permission, he said he was excited to scan a pregnancy, as it was a stage he rarely got to see. And there it was. A teeny, tiny shape, already with a clearly formed head and body and four little stumps that would grow to become his limbs. And a heartbeat. My heart beat fiercely in my chest as I watched the tiny white dot pulsate on the screen. My baby's heart was beating clearly. Our scan clearly showed a viable pregnancy, in fact it clearly showed our baby and more than that, it showed me what a truly wonderful and talented man our wonderful Professor Killick was.

That was now three years ago and our lives had changed so much since then. It was lovely to see Prof again, tell him about our little boy and without hesitation he suggested to try Clomid for a second time.

What I remember most clearly about our visits to the clinic was that each time, whilst they gave us drugs and advice, what they mostly gave us was hope. We would park the car each time in nervous anticipation and yet each time, no matter what the outcome of tests or progress reviews, we always left with hearts full of hope. I can wholly understand how many IVF babies come to be named Hope or Faith because you must have both in abundance to survive the journey. Hull IVF Clinic used to readily give us both on each visit.

For six months I took the Clomid without success and a second visit to the clinic resulted in another six month prescription. Whilst there is a specific time each month that you obviously focus on in terms of whether your period arrives, when you are trying for a baby you actually live your life fortnight by fortnight. At day 14 of your cycle you are deemed most fertile as you ovulate. From day 11 to 17 you are therefore advised to have sex as much as possible to increase your chances of conceiving. You can buy ovulation tests that indicate when you are actually ovulating which are also supposed to help. Each month

I would attend the clinic on day 21 to check my Progesterone levels ensuring the Clomid was indeed stimulating my ovaries. And so, month after month, we planned, we tested, we did 'it' and we waited to see if we'd been successful. On and on, round and round, the cycle went like a non-stop merry-go-round. We bought ovulation sticks, ovulation kits, pregnancy tests, you name it, if it was marketed to assist fertility we bought it!

As soon as my period would start, I'd gasp, cry, then take a deep breath and work out my next cycle and when I'd be ovulating next. It seems mechanical, and it is. Some say it is loveless, but that's never a feeling we had. Despite the planning, sometimes the sex on nights we may have preferred just to sleep, we promised each other that we'd always ensure any baby would be conceived with love. Of course there were times for both of us when we'd like a night off, or just didn't feel like being passionate, there were nights when I'd literally drag myself off my pillow but we knew there was a small window each month and so each month we had to give it our best shot.

Even Jason, the hot blooded bloke in the relationship, had times when even he couldn't muster the enthusiasm but we constantly talked about how we both felt and were both reassured that it was more to do with the forced timing of the activity rather than our desire for each other. I can wholly understand how switching your sex life on and off like a light switch, for an outcome being something other than simply pleasure, could put a strain on a relationship but for us, despite sometimes needing more coaxing than usual each time, it brought us closer and overall, we had a great time!

The best times however were those few days after my period had finished but before there was any chance of me ovulating. Those few days when it didn't matter what we did, I probably wouldn't get pregnant anyway and there was no chance I could actually be pregnant so there was no nervous waiting to find out either. We had fun and we loved loving each other with all the spontaneity any normal relationship should have. We relaxed, we could be our old selves and we loved each other fully, in our own way, on our own terms and it was uplifting.

Eleven months later and there was still no sign.

Is time running out?

I went to the clinic for yet another of my monthly Day 21 blood tests and sat alone in the waiting room waiting for the nurse. I had one week left until my period was due then one final month's worth of Clomid remaining. So that would have been twelve months on Clomid and still no success.

It was starting to dawn on us that the drug wasn't working. I fell pregnant with Zac on my fourth cycle, so why wasn't it working this time? I had two more chances and then our only next option would be IVF. I guess I'd known it was a possibility that I would need IVF, but I'd never really considered that would be a path I'd be going on. Waiting for my appointment, I started to look round the waiting room. Posters, leaflets and booklets offering advice and counselling were everywhere plastered on all the walls. I'd seen them countless times before but for some reason this time they were more than wall coverings, I was actually reading them and taking in what they said. This suddenly became a real situation and a terrifying one at that.

A noticeboard proudly displayed the clinic's success statistics. The team currently had the best record in Europe for the first six months of the year and briefly I was immensely proud of them, they deserved it. But the statistic wasn't 100%; they didn't create a child for everyone. Attending the clinic didn't bring certainty and for many people, they will have undergone many cycles of treatment and yet still they were without a child.

Whilst full of hope, IVF was also terrifying to me. It wasn't the copious drugs, pain or invasive procedures that bothered me, but as I saw it, IVF was like the great white knight. After months of stimulation drugs, I saw IVF as my last resort, my all conquering saviour and whilst I had yet to start the treatment, it was always still there as another potential chance, an option, hope. Once I started down that route, there was of course a chance it wouldn't work, that I would be one of those statistics of couples who were unsuccessful and then what would I do? I couldn't face the thought that I'd cash in my great white knight and it wouldn't come good for me. I felt better knowing I had that option still left in the locker and I wasn't sure I was ready to risk that chance just yet. As I got nearer to the end of my Clomid, this thought that I'd been burying deep within me for months now suddenly overwhelmed me.

My eyes pricked. I suddenly felt them sting and as I blinked, a tear ran down my cheek. To this day I still don't know why it happened on that day but I had what I could only best describe as a meltdown. I started crying uncontrollably in the waiting room. I tried and tried to pull it back, to get a grip, but I couldn't stop the sobs.

I had no tissues and couldn't see any in the waiting room. I couldn't sit there any more with tears literally pouring down my face. I went to the reception window and as Roxanne slid back the glass screen, through my desperate gasps I asked for a tissue. They quickly whisked round to the waiting room and ushered me into one of the consultation rooms. I cried and cried and was simply unable to stop the sobs. The enormity of the realisation that I really was struggling to conceive and that perhaps one day I might run out of options and may never have another child, hit me that day with the force of a ton of bricks.

The nurses tried to console me and talk to me as they took my blood for the day 21 test, but I could only apologise as I tried to convince them that I was fine and explain that I had no idea where all the tears and emotion had suddenly come from. Obviously they had seen it all before but to me, at that time, I literally thought they'd think I was some sort of nutter.

I made my way out towards the car park and sat in the car for five minutes or so. Tears were still flowing. It almost made me laugh but all I could think was that I'd only popped out from work saying I'd be half an hour. I'd have to stop the tears somehow. How could I walk back into the office in this sorry state?

I called one of my best friends Jo. Jo and I are to each other, the big and little sisters neither of us ever had. We've been there for each other all our lives and in many ways have shared similar experiences and have been able to support each other. She was the one I'd ask those awkward questions during my teenage years, the one who I'd learn the songs to Wham with despite the fact she always insisted she was the one to marry George Michael and for as long as I can remember she has always been the one who has bought the same items of clothing or gifts or treats as me, despite never having spoken about them! Regardless blood, DNA and parentage, she has always been my big sister in every sense and I love her dearly.

Strangely, or perhaps not so, she too had undergone IVF and so as well as being able to understand a lot of how I felt at that time, she could also decipher a lot of the lingo they used in the clinic and helped me make sense of the advice I was often given.

"Where are you?, Can you talk" I stuttered. "I'm in Tesco, but yeh sure I can talk, are you OK?" I hated it when she sounded worried about me but I was struggling to put on a brave face for her that day.

"I've just had a complete meltdown in the IVF clinic and I've been crying for half an hour and I still can't stop!"

"Oh my God, I bet that was dead embarrassing!" That was all she said but she'd done it. I laughed out loud! She made me laugh at a time when laughing felt so far away from what I was feeling. There are few people who would have or could have got away with saying that at that time, but it was perfect and just what I needed. Of course we talked some more and I cried some more but a new sense of grounding had taken hold and after another half hour I was able to put my face back on and get back to work. My big sis had once again got me through a crisis.

The fact that I had broken down did highlight just how worried and frustrated I was getting as the weeks whizzed by and the drugs ran out. Perhaps we'd left it too late to start trying again and had missed the opportunity based on the theory that it was easier to conceive once you'd had a baby. Perhaps we'd left it too late to have another child full stop. I'd longed for a baby and we'd been blessed with Zac and maybe one baby was all we were destined to have. Maybe we had asked, we had received and that was it. It should have been enough.

Deciding to seek help from the clinic was simple, getting the drugs prescribed was easy and I suppose I thought I'd get caught just as quick, or if not in 4 months like last time then, 6 or at least 8 maybe.

Feeling Raw

The most ridiculous thing anyone can ever say to someone trying for a baby is "try to relax and try not to think about it". You could never ever realise what a waste of breath it is to say that unless you have been in that position. Theoretically, whilst there may be some truth in the statement, it is impossible to put into practice. You may as well say "don't draw breath when you get up in the morning!"

Rubbing salt into an open wound is a good metaphor to describe what it's like, going about your normal day when everything around you seems to remind you of your pain at not being able to get pregnant. It sounds dramatic but honestly, I got to the point where I couldn't get through a single day without the feeling that something was stabbing me in the chest.

I knew Jason longed for a baby as I did; of course he did and was as committed to our efforts as I was. But I was also aware that he didn't suffer each day as I did, didn't have the same feelings of grief or frustration as I did and couldn't believe it sometimes when I explained my rambling thoughts to him about the specific pain I'd felt on a particular day. I'm 100% convinced that this is down to the 'men are from Mars and women are from Venus' theory and that him being a man, whilst loving, sensitive and supportive, meant that his frustrations were less frequent and only caused by the more obvious triggers.

For me, it was everywhere, every day. Every birthday meant I was another year older meaning reduced chance of conceiving and my being an older mother to my children. Zac's passing birthdays really hurt, as he became 3 and then 4 and so did the specific month passing each year that was the cut off that even if I did conceive I wouldn't have the baby before Zac's next birthday. The gap between him and my would-be children was widening month by month.

There were so many dates, so many milestones that cut through my heart and hurt like hell. I was constantly calculating the age gap, what school years they'd be in and with every family milestone that passed I'd be considering whether I would have had a baby by the next or worse still, that I should have had a baby by the next. Birthdays, holidays, Christmas, anniversaries, you name it, each milestone that passed, hurt that little bit more.

My cousin Paula had her baby girl Zoe just two weeks after I had Zac. We'd both tried for years and then to have our children just a fortnight apart and both be called three letter names beginning with 'Z' meant we were always destined to be closer than we'd ever been before. We vowed to keep the kids close and ensure they saw as much of each other as possible, despite living at opposite ends of the M62.

Zac and Zoe were double trouble, terrific friends and loved each other dearly despite being so young. When they were two and a half, Paula had a second daughter Elin, my lovely, sweet God-daughter. Elin was a gorgeous baby with the most beautiful big brown eyes that just melted you when you looked down into them. With Zac and Zoe being so close, the desire to have another child close to Elin's age was immense and every time we'd meet up and I'd see Elin getting older, looking into her big brown eyes would only remind me how time was passing and I still hadn't produced a cousin for her to play with.

Zac had a lot of friends, in particular a gorgeous little girl across the road, Giselle. Giselle was the youngest of three girls, who were all terrific playing with and caring for Zac. At 7 months older than Zac, Giselle was obviously ahead of him in terms of development in their early years but with older siblings nurturing and encouraging her, she often seemed far more advanced. Dainty and blonde, she had a feather-like body that disguised her feisty nature! She could put anyone in his or her place and often did!

Our house was at the end of a cul-de-sac, so it was fairly safe for the children to play out but we still felt Zac was too young to play out in the front without us. Often, if we were doing jobs in the house or the back garden, he would look out of the front windows at Giselle riding up and down the street with her older sisters looking after her. The strong unit of three sisters, playing with each other and bringing each other on used to sadden me when I'd look at my child, playing inside on his own. Don't get me wrong; Zac was by no means a child who went without or who had a poor childhood. Certainly not. But to see the joy that brothers and sisters gave other children, a joy I had known myself with my brother, only sought to make me more determined he should have a sibling.

Zac had made a best friend at nursery almost from the time they could crawl towards each other. Harry and Zac were hilarious together and were inseparable. Harry had just turned 2 when his baby sister Millie was born and he was very proud of her. At 2, the boys started to say a few words and as Millie grew, they would both talk about her, more and more. Whenever Zac saw her he was so gentle towards her, crouching to stroke her cheek and help her with whatever she was doing. He was so lovely around her, so caring, I couldn't wait for him to have a baby sister himself.

My friend's children were also a painful trigger as they grew up quickly and reminded me that the gulf between their children and mine was growing. Most of our best friends all had their children close together and out of five couples, they had 10 children within five years of each other and it was great to see them all playing when we'd get together on holidays or weekend barbecues.

I remember telling my friend Claire that she should wait for me, when having her second baby as I was trying too. "Hang on for me" I used to joke. Her eldest Charlie was three when Harry came along but it was still another three years before Zac finally arrived. Whilst the boys played with Zac, he was clearly so much younger than them and as they grew into much bigger boys, the gap between them and my would-be second child just grew and grew. For some reason that mattered to me. That my children wouldn't be the friends of my friends seemed to really get under my skin and upset me. Of course it didn't matter, it still doesn't matter today, but to me, it was a huge injustice and massive frustration. I'm sure the core of that frustration was the fact that it wasn't down to any decision I'd taken, but it really used to sadden me.

I'd watch other neighbours' children playing, two brothers and one boy, an only child. Of course they all got on well, but it would literally feel like my heart was breaking to see the young boy on his own when the brothers had gone in for tea, or to see him wandering back home having been turned away from their house when they weren't allowed to play out. I never had reason to think he felt lonely, or that he felt isolated in any way as they always looked like they had enormous fun. I never spoke to his Mum or to him to know whether he did indeed feel any loneliness, yet knowing my child didn't have a sibling to fall back on, rely on, play with when nobody else was playing out, used to fill me with horror and dread. In reality, I knew it wouldn't be the end of the world, but it wasn't what I wanted and the fact that it was out of my control was probably the catalyst for this fear as well as the frustration.

Brotherly love

Enriching Zac's life was a huge part of why we wanted another child. Two friends, one who was an only child himself and another who had made the decision to just have her son, had both talked to me about the virtues of having one child. How they felt life could and had made up for not having a sibling, in so many other ways. More focus, more quality time, no sharing or competing for attention and I'm sure more material objects or additional opportunities that more money allowed.

Both gave me another perspective and definitely something to think about. Neither felt they missed out and both felt they had either had an enriched life or had provided a rich and fulfilling life for their child. I have no reason to think otherwise, both are sensible people and both are loving individuals with very happy families.

I have to say that I don't just have rose-tinted glasses on family life or siblings. I am very, very fortunate to have a very loving family and a fabulous relationship with my brother. Andrew is 3 years younger than me. We were both active, outdoor-loving children. We ran everywhere, went on endless bike rides and would play in the fields at the end of our road for hours and hours with all the neighbours' kids. We had a free and easy childhood. When we were younger however, we often also fought like cat and dog. On one occasion when Andrew wanted to plug his Spectrum computer into the TV I was watching, we spent more than an hour fighting, which resulted in me throwing the keyboard at him and cutting his hand open. Another time, he actually broke his wrist after I had raised my knees to defend myself against the series of punches he was throwing at me, as I lay on the sofa in the space he wanted! Another trip to casualty!

But it was all just the usual kids scrapping and besides that, we got on pretty well. For some reason I'd always felt protective of my little brother, who soon grew to be my much bigger little brother. He struggled more academically whereas I found learning relatively easy by comparison and I'd often sneakily help him with homework, as I couldn't bear to see him struggle or be upset. It was probably when I left to go to university that our relationship really forged the strong bond that we still have today. We missed each other hugely and whilst we were getting on with our lives as they took us in new directions, meeting new friends and enjoying new experiences, the distance definitely made us grow fonder of each other.

At 21, Andrew took off on a trip around the world on his own. I'd never known anyone actually take at year out and travel the world at that time and to think of my little brother doing it was utterly terrifying, especially on his own! The night before he left I had the most heart wrenching pain in my chest that I couldn't sleep and had to get up. I was absolutely terrified that I'd never see him again. That this was it, he would go and he'd be foolish enough to try something daring and never come home. I typed a short letter telling him I loved him so much, was so proud of him and begged him to promise me he wouldn't do anything stupid. I also realised that night that out of all the millions of people in the world, there was in fact only 2 people who had been born from exactly the same place, our Mum, and that was him and I. From that night I have never forgotten that fact. (I should say that after landing in his first stop, Bombay of all places, he called to say he'd arrived safely and promptly told me off for sneaking the note into his bag, as having tried to be brave in saying goodbye to us all at the airport, he promptly found and read the note and was in tears before the plane even took off!)

We also shared a huge love for our Mum. Dad left when I was in my mid teens in a fairly acrimonious divorce, one that left me severing all ties with him when I was 18. In those days, Mum was our rock, our anchor, the woman who gave us never-ending love and affection and who struggled but succeeded to continue to provide a warm and loving home for the two of us. Our trio had an "us against the world" mentality and often, when called to the Poll Tax office to explain our unpaid bills, that was actually the reality.

There was never ever a time that I can remember when she didn't make us feel that we were her number one priority and I do think that one important lesson she taught us was that you should love and support your family, without question. I do believe this rubbed off on both Andrew and I, as over the years the three of us have always been there for each other, offering unwavering love and constant support and where possible, Andrew and I have tried to repay her earlier efforts and sacrifices wherever we can.

As a result, since our late teens, Andrew and I have been exceptionally close and I know I am very lucky to have such a fantastic relationship. I cannot imagine not having had him in my life, despite the occasional scrap! I know not all sibling relationships are like this and I know that Mum is largely responsible for the nurturing of this closeness but to have the opportunity to give Zac the joy that I know of having a brother, or indeed a sister, was something I dearly wanted.

And yet, others viewed it all differently. The friend I mentioned, who was an only child, was approaching 50. He felt he'd had a great life and was completely fulfilled, but as he pointed out, his parents decided not to try for any more and all their focus had been on him. Right up until his beloved father passed away he had a terrific loving relationship with both parents and knew no different. He has never known what it's like to have a sibling and therefore doesn't feel he's missed out.

I don't know the reason why my other friend I mentioned, with the one child, decided that one was enough, but I do know that she did make the conscious decision. From the moment she had to arrange for an expanding waistband on her work uniform, she has loved her little boy and now as he is a teenager, she feels she has been able to give him so much more in terms of holidays, experiences and her time than she could have done if she'd had two or more.

I can understand the sense, in fact of course it makes sense on a practical level, but it also makes a huge difference whether you have made that decision yourself or whether the decision to have just one child is made for you. If I decided that actually, I thought Zac deserved everything I could possibly provide for him; a private education maybe, holidays to Dubai and Disney or my 100% focus and that I could only provide all that if I didn't have any more children, then of course my entire outlook would be different.

But that was never the case. Zac, I knew, would hopefully always feel fulfilled, even if he ended up with 10 siblings, but being part of a bigger family, with a brother or sister, or both, in my mind was the best thing possible that I could provide for him. The fact that Zac was still our only child was most certainly not our decision at that time and that was why it hurt so much.

Our only child

Several times it did cross my mind that maybe we were destined to have only one child. Zac was growing into a wonderfully independent little boy, he was good at amusing himself in his playroom with his toy figures, cars or running around outside with his football.

He had a vibrant personality but would often be quite shy in front of other people. At home he was the life and soul, in fact often boisterous, but amongst our friends, even those he knew really well, he was quite timid and took time to warm up and come round.

He was very thoughtful and caring. He'd often ask quite a meaningful question about something that happened weeks before that he'd obviously been contemplating or on the very rare occasion he'd catch me crying, he'd hold me close when I was putting him to bed and ask: "Mummy why were you crying?"

Whilst 2007 was a tremendously happy year with the arrival of Zac it would also prove to be the start of what would turn out to be one of the biggest economic recessions the world had known. Little did we know at that time that in the very next few months in 2008, whilst bringing many joyful moments with our new baby, our family would be flung into one of the most stressful times we'll hopefully ever have to endure.

The Thursday before I was due to start back at work on the Monday after my maternity leave, my business partner, who had been the main funder in our business, told me there was no money to pay me. There is no gain for this book in discussing what went on because the whole scenario and how it was handled broke my heart, suffice to say we were one of the first families we knew of to experience the 'credit crunch' as it became known, and almost overnight I lost my business, my income, my direction and someone I loved who I thought was my friend.

With more and more people starting to feel the pinch, the motor industry started to slow down and as a trader, the job became harder and harder for Jason. Worse still, we'd invested in a commercial property venture to try to do our best for the family and maximise our savings, but with this investment being made on the back of us thinking we had stable jobs and now a crisis in the property market, our family's future was suddenly, massively at risk.

I'm pleased to say, we stuck in there, worked our asses off, cut right back on everything and we survived. But the fear never left us. We continue to this day to have an underlying desire to have our cash around us, have an accessible nest egg, and live life well within our means. We're not flash or extravagant and whilst some might say we are relatively well off, we know how easily it can all fall away.

It was on the backdrop of this experience that made us wonder about how much more we could give Zac if it indeed was meant to be that he would be our only child. As we don't live in the immediate catchment for the local comprehensive I'd like him to attend, private school would be a possible option. Having attended a great comprehensive and done relatively well academically, I've always been of the belief that the money I'd save by not sending my children to private school would be best spent giving them great experiences I could afford more comfortably. Those rocky months certainly made me think differently about how life would be if we did have more children and whether or not it would cripple us financially and put life as we currently knew it at risk. Could we actually afford more children? We had many a sleepless night wondering if we were going to lose the roof above our heads and I was buying the bare essentials and basic food supplies to fill our bellies and yet here I was considering bringing another mouth to feed and clothe into our home! Those thoughts were real but fleeting. They were a worry but they were also quickly put to the back of my mind as I had to believe if it was meant to be, we would, as we always had done, find a way to care for our family.

I don't know if it was "only child syndrome" or just in my make up, but at that time I was absolutely Zac obsessed. When we took someone on at work I'd always have to warn them that I talked about my little boy a lot and apologised in advance for the daily stories they'd have to hear about what he'd been up to!

He started introducing imaginary friends into the family. Roger, Kenny and Harry were frequently round at our house playing football, eating dinner with us and one day, even holding up story time at Nursery whilst "Roger went to the toilet"! Zac's imagination knew no bounds and frequently had us in stitches. He'd often talk about Roger's little boy or baby Harry, and then he introduced baby Jessica and baby Tilly. Jason and I were obviously super sensitive about it but it was also lovely to see his caring, nurturing side develop, even though he was still on his own.

I knew that whilst the practical side of me sometimes suggested I could perhaps give more to just Zac if he remained our only child, every other fibre in my body told me that I should keep trying to give him a brother or sister. I'd often just look at him and think how unfair it was, wonder what he'd be like as a big brother or simply grit my teeth in irritation that it hadn't happened yet.

I'd never really understood the term 'maternal instinct' before. As a young girl, I never thought I felt it, though I loved young children and was surrounded by younger cousins. Feeling maternal was something I thought unambitious, lentil-eating, home-loving girls felt and yet, when you want a child and are in a situation where you aren't getting pregnant, I can only imagine that the undeniable, strong urge to get pregnant or hold your new baby is that very maternal instinct expressing itself through Mother Nature. I felt it all right. I hadn't purposefully turned it on, or requested that feeling. It was just there; all the time and nothing was making it go away. It was in my head, in my heart and at times I even felt it in my aching arms. It was all consuming, in my daydreaming or in my thoughts at the most inopportune moments, disturbing a more serious chain of thought.

Team Davies, as we three often called ourselves, was also extremely close and we'd often be honest with Zac about what was going on in our lives. Obviously this was a subject that even Jason and I couldn't explain so we never dared open up the box of questions that any suggestion of trying for another baby might pose if we talked to Zac about it. I found it really hard not to talk to him about what we were going through though. I felt dishonest in some ways that he wasn't part of it all or we were keeping something from him. It sounds silly when he wasn't much more than a baby himself, but the three of us were such a close unit and sometimes I felt terribly dishonest for keeping such a big, important secret from him.

It was like that feeling sometimes where you feel something is written all over your face, even though nobody has really any idea about what is going on in your life, your head or your heart. It felt like he knew something was going on, somehow knew I was unhappy and that there was something terribly important going on in our lives but he was unaware what it was. That was often a seemingly ridiculous sounding feeling but a real, hurtful one none-the-less. I suppose it was just yet another example of the irrational thoughts and feelings that this less than normal situation created.

When he asked if we were ever going to have a baby, I'd carry on the conversation and talk it through with him as I'd vowed never to shut him down or change the subject. I wanted him to be aware that it was a possibility, but just not get his heart set on it. I was always aware that I'd need to introduce the idea as I wanted to avoid him being jealous at such at time should another child eventually come along. I'd ask what he'd call a new baby, would he help look after it and make a joke about him changing nappies. I'd always end with, "well we'll see what happens, hopefully we will one day, we'll all just have to keep being good boys and girls and maybe we'll be lucky enough." Whilst this line of response seemed to work well, I dreaded the day he might ask if we hadn't had another baby because we'd not been a good boy or girl.

Frequently I also desperately wanted to explain to him just how hard I was trying and that actually it wasn't as easy as going to Tesco and just buying another baby! I wanted to tell him that we wanted it too and for him to know Mummy and Daddy were really, really trying hard to get one. Sadly, I guess it was also growing more and more important and worrying for me that Zac may think there was something wrong with his Mummy, or that I had let him down in some way, but thankfully this silly thought would only rear its head in my more darker moments.

Hurting every day

With anything in life, when you suddenly become aware of a new subject, topic or emotion, it seems there is a reminder everywhere, right in front of your eyes, from that moment onwards. If you meet someone for the first time, who works for a particular company you've never heard of before, you can guarantee you will see that company's vans, adverts or uniforms everywhere thereafter.

Reminders of my inability to conceive were very much like that. Everywhere, every day, rearing their ugly head when I'd least expect. The constant reminders were completely unavoidable. I'm certain it was simply because I was acutely sensitive but everywhere around there seemed to be babies and bumps. It often felt like Mums with babies, pregnant girls or parents with prams were actually making a beeline for me, just to make sure I noticed them. Sometimes in more lighter moments, I'd walk through a shopping centre or the centre of town and play a game with myself to walk and try to avoid a pram or pregnant young girl and then feel like they were aiming for me like some sort of computer game. At those more tolerable, light-hearted times, I could see it for what it all was, just typical life, a busy shopping centre and my over-sensitivity. Of course they weren't targeting me or tormenting me, but in my more sensitive, irrational and uncontrollably sad times I could have fallen to my knees with the enormity of the pain that the sight of seemingly so many mums or tums would stir in me. Lunch breaks in town were often too painful to bother taking.

And yet, it was often those close to me, friends, family or colleagues, who could often hurt me more. Of course, many had no idea at all how much their words would affect me and undoubtedly would be mortified if they realised.

There were regularly questions that I'm sure form part of basic conversations between friends every day and yet, at that time, they would tear me apart. Often they were probably spat out as just fillers when friends or acquaintances couldn't think of anything else to say: "You having any more?", "Isn't it about time you popped another one out?" or "You thought about having any more yet?". For a while I was unaffected and simply replied, "well yes, perhaps we'll see, you never know", but the longer the wait went on, the more unable I was to brush the questions aside and smile. I think it must be how you answer accusations when you are in fact guilty of what you're being accused of. When something is on your mind so acutely and is so sensitive and important, you simply can't just brush a question off and any reply you make seems forced and clumsy.

It seemed like we had hit a milestone in Zac's development where suddenly there was a green light above our heads that invited people to question where the next child was, or indeed, more hurtful, why we hadn't had the next child yet.

Then there were the questions that sent a flare up to warn me that the "You having any more?" question was on its way. They'd ask, "So how old is he?" or "Gosh isn't he growing?" and my heart would sink…wait. …wait for it…. it's coming… I could feel the next killer question coming and the anger and hurt would start to rise up in me, as I'd try to prepare myself. Sometimes I'd hear myself saying "here we go, armour on, get ready, please try not to be cross when it comes, try your hardest not to show how much it hurts!" On these occasions I'd really, really try not to be defensive or objectionable, but it was often difficult. Timing was everything. If I had just had a period or a negative test or simply been out for a sandwich and seen a 'baby on board' suction sign on the back of a car, it would obviously be the worst time to ask. There were times during each month when the pain was so acute and subject so raw, that to have someone pry into it, used to ignite a fury I could barely hide.

One time at the start of a regular monthly meeting, a client casually asked how my family was and how my little boy was doing. Enjoying the banter before the real stuff started, I was happy to reply that Zac was fine, growing fast and funny as ever. His next question changed all that. In fact, it wasn't actually the next question of "have you thought about having any more" which in itself is fairly innocent; it was the series of more personal, thoughtless questions that followed that really changed the mood. It was a targeted barrage of relentless quizzing and I struggled to deflect the unwanted attention.

"It's about time you had another isn't it?", "Have you tried for any more", "Most people only leave it for 2 or 3 years until they have another, what is he 4? you're leaving it a bit late aren't you?". He was a client, there were others in the room and we had a meeting about his forthcoming marketing to get through, so standing up, screaming at him and slapping his face was not really an option open to me. I tried to bring forward the feeling of pity at his ignorance that was stirring somewhere deep inside me. What a pig. It worked to some degree, well at least to keep me in my seat long enough to muster a shrug and a non-committal, dismissive response, then quickly change the subject. It put a dampener on yet another day but it was sadly a dark mood change I had been getting used to.

Another time, I remember I was talking to a supplier at work whose wife had just found out she was pregnant and at first I'd been really pleased for them as they were a lovely couple. Though I had just two months left of my Clomid, I could still appreciate that others would still experience the joy of finding out they were expecting and having known that myself three years earlier, I could still find myself being delighted knowing how they felt. This however, all turned sour. He began to explain how they'd planned to have the baby to coincide with school holidays so that his wife, a teacher, could have extended maternity leave using the summer holidays. They'd tried once, conceived and their plan was in action. I was, of course, astounded and dismayed at their unbelievable luck but this turned into anger when he rounded off his boast with: "Innit about time you popped another out? You wanna get on with it!"

I couldn't get my head round his sheer ignorance and complacency at how they had got pregnant so easily and for thinking that it should be the same for everyone else. Of course, when you haven't had experience of infertility you simply do believe that you just have sex and hey presto, nine months later out pops a baby. In fact, I myself had spent years being terrified and utterly convinced that I would definitely fall pregnant following a ripped condom or impulsive lustful moment so why wouldn't others think that it really was that simple too?

I should have been more understanding but I was reeling in a mix of surprise, anger, frustration and deep, deep hurt and without thinking I blurted out: "I can't have any more!!!" I shocked myself! It was wrong, really wrong of me to say that and to this day I'm ashamed of myself because at that time, I didn't know that that was the case at all. I can only explain it by saying I just wanted to lash out, to hurt him in some way as he'd hurt me, but I immediately deeply regretted saying it.

Another good friend deeply upset me when we were on holiday in Portugal. At two, Zac was still quite shy but he was more so on this particular day as we'd been on holiday on our own for a week before more than 20 of our friends came out to join us for a wedding and on their first afternoon, most of them had joined us on the beach. I'm sure my poor baby didn't know what the hell was going on after a quiet family week and then such a mass arrival. Understandably he stayed close to our sides and wasn't keen on playing with anyone else.

"What he needs is a brother or sister to bring him out of himself!" said our friend. If someone has ever said anything to you that has made you feel like you've had a knife through the heart then you'll know exactly what effect his words had on me. I said nothing. I didn't know what to say. I knew what I wanted to say, but to do that would have created a terrible atmosphere and hurt our friend in a way that was totally unfair. Inside I was screaming at him partly that he had no idea how much I did want another child for Zac to play with and partly that it was he who had in fact frightened my child so bloody much in the first place! He never normally paid Zac any attention so that when he did, of course my poor baby was going to be shy! It was certainly not because he was an only child! He could never have known how hurtful his words were, how much I desperately wanted to give my boy a brother or sister or how offended I was at his apparent criticism of my child.

One particularly offending comment was from my hairdresser who was pursuing a line of questioning over and over about why I hadn't had another child, which finished with: "Your fella got no lead in his pencil or what?" Criticise me, that's one thing, but criticise my family and that is a whole different matter. I was incensed. Without a care for the atmosphere it would inevitably create and without thought that he had a pair of sharp scissors in his hands, I hissed back that he should keep his mouth shut about things he knew nothing about and not dare comment on my family ever again. After composing myself, a second later I added that it was nothing to do with Jason, for fear my outburst may have indicated otherwise! It was a silent and swift trim and blow-dry after that!

Such painful experiences proved to be an important lesson in life however. After being put into some extremely uncomfortable and often hurtful situations, I now know how hard it can be to be quizzed on such a subject, even if the questions are asked in all innocence. Now, I would never ever ask anyone if they were trying or thinking about having a child. I would hate to make someone feel how I have often felt on the receiving end of an apparently innocent question.

And yet, I am sure there are other questions I've asked people that have hurt them, without me knowing or meaning any harm. I may have asked someone if they're getting married without knowing they desperately want to but their boyfriend doesn't and I may have unintentionally, yet deeply upset them. I knew people didn't mean anything by their questions to me. That's just life. You just don't know what is really going on in people's lives or how your words can potentially hurt them. And yet, despite knowing that, it never took the sting out of their words.

Pressures from a toddler

Zac was starting to understand where babies come from. Not in the biblical, physical sense, thank goodness, but that other families had babies in their houses and that, in simplistic terms, they originally came from Mummies' tummies. Fortunately, having had a caesarean 'sunroof' job with Zac, I was able to show him my scar on my tummy and explain that's where he popped out, so avoided any awkward questions about where babies actually came from and how they were made!

His questions were however getting more and more frequent and in depth. His nursery key workers often told us how gentle and caring he was with the younger children, and how he loved to help the grown ups by fetching toys or dummies for all the babies. He was becoming more aware of babies all around him and as more new babies appeared in the baby room, with some being the younger brothers or sisters of his friends, his questions become more direct.

With the innocence of a three year old, they were obvious questions, but when they came out of the blue or were randomly dropped into a conversation we were having about which dessert to have, they often knocked Jason and I off our feet!

"When are we getting a baby?", "Why is our baby not here yet?", "Where will our baby come from?".

Zac would sometimes talk about Millie, the little sister of his best friend Harry and just as he would ask for a football kit or a Fireman Sam figure like Harry, he was obviously wondering whether he was going to get a baby sister like Harry too. He'd often fuss Millie whenever we'd see her. He would always rub her cheek or go to give her a hug. He'd rush to help if he saw she had dropped something and would always talk about the times he'd seen her in the baby room during the day. It was often difficult to explain why Harry had a sister and he didn't but it was an easier conversation to have when I could distract him with questions back at him about what he had seen her doing that day. He always had a tale to tell and forget his original enquiry. It was only afterwards, when I had time to reflect alone and I could let my guard down, that his questions really hit home and I'd allow myself to feel upset.

As we grew closer to starting the IVF treatment it seemed his questions became more direct, and sometimes I even felt, somewhat prophetic. He'd always talk about 'the baby', and annoyingly, I'd allowed myself to feel comfortable with the expression as if it brought some reality to the situation. He used the term and he lead the questions, but often I used to have to give my head a shake as it was almost as if I found comfort in the conversation. I was perhaps allowing myself to believe it was all real. He'd ask inquisitive questions like "Was the baby in your tummy when I was in there too Mummy?" or more practical queries that were obviously concerning him such as "Can the baby sleep in my room when it comes?"

Despite feeling some warm hope with our little chats, I was always 100% careful in what I said to him and to manage his expectations. I used to listen to him talking and be saying to myself "you need to be careful Helen for his sake, you're desperate, not stupid." He was obviously far too young to understand the complete picture and any false hope given to such a young boy could be shattering later.

We did however say our prayers together and sometimes pray for a new baby. Brought up a Catholic, I always felt my faith had done well to keep me on the straight and narrow. Going to church every Sunday had given me an acute sense that there was someone listening to your prayers and that you should always be sincerely thankful for any blessing you received. Though not devout nor strict, my faith was still important and there were elements such as prayer and thanksgiving that I wanted to bestow on Zac to help guide him.

"Please God, could we please have a new baby. We promise to love it and care for it. Thank you for our loving family and thank you for listening to our prayers."..........And then a little voice would say "and can we have two babies, a boy and a girl and can the baby boy be good at football?" His prayers were lovely to hear, funny yet serious!

My Granma and Mum were both loyal to their Catholic faith. Amazingly, after having one and a half ovaries removed when she was just 19, my mum managed to conceive both my brother and I with just half an ovary, with no medical assistance. Every time I stopped to think about that amazing fact, especially in the situation I was in with my want for children, I couldn't help but wonder how truly miraculous it is that Andrew and I are here at all.

The month before I conceived Zac, my Mum gave me a prayer card and medal dedicated to St Gerard, the patron saint of motherhood. Her mother, my Granma, had given it her when she was trying for me. I immediately treasured it. It meant a lot that Mum had had it close to her when trying for me, but it was extra special knowing that the original intention had been made by my beloved Granma.

I put the card and medal under my pillow and said the prayer on the card every night, without fail, before I went to sleep. To realise the timing, in that I fell pregnant with Zac soon after it was given to me was made extra special, not just because I'd was finally pregnant but to think that there was some link to both my Mum and Grandma and that we shared something special. St Gerard became one of my most cherished possessions.

Sometime later, Jo was trying for a child and I gave her St Gerard and asked them both to look after each other (in fact I told her in no uncertain terms not to bloody lose him!). When she told me she was pregnant, my love for and belief in my St Gerard medal grew stronger.

He remained by the side of my bed and a few times, Zac had seen him and asked what it was and who the man was in the picture. On one occasion I explained that he looked after all Mummies in the world and sometimes, if they are good, he gives them babies. I never thought any more about it. Months later, out of the blue Zac said something and I couldn't make out what he was trying to say. "SaynDewar!"? He was now getting to the age where he'd get frustrated if we didn't understand him and would sometimes give up trying to say the words but give us clues instead. "You know, that man in your room who is going to give us a baby!" Ah SaynDewar was Saint Gerard!!

Another time Zac had been snuggling in our bed before going to his own bed and was dragging out the time, trying every stalling tactic in the book to avoid leaving. "Kiss for Mummy, kiss for Daddy…and kiss for SaynDewar" He leant over, grabbed my St Gerard medal and kissed it, as he'd probably seen me do many times. That night, Zac slept in our bed all night. He'd pulled a blinder! He knew all my buttons to press!

Zac's quizzes about babies were obviously occasionally tricky for me to deal with, but more often than not they were refreshing and his innocence and directness would remind me what a blessing this little boy really was for Jason and I and how lucky we were to have such a fabulous child already.

On one occasion when he was asking about how you got a baby, I had answered that I had to be a really, really good girl and if I could keep it up, then I might be lucky enough to get a baby in my tummy. I was sat on the floor in front of my tall mirror doing my make up and Zac, as usual was sat in the middle of my crossed legs. After a few moments he leapt up and said, "I know Mummy! If you don't shout at me, you'll be a good girl, then you'll get a baby!" At three years old, he was wise beyond his years and as well as howl laughing at his delight at possibly working the situation to his advantage, I also felt a pang of regret that my boy was obviously trying desperately to think of ways to make it alright. If it was at all ever possible, I loved him a little more at that moment, for making me laugh so hysterically and for caring enough to come up with a plan.

Zac's growing inquisitiveness, his youthful honesty, his absolute innocence and his own obvious desire to have a new baby in the family were all beautiful, lovely qualities for us to witness develop. Yet at the same time in their own way, they were so painful at times to have to deal with. They were constant reminders. They put a sort of realism on my desire in how a new baby could positively impact his life. More than any of that, to know that he too wanted a baby brother or sister, to either have someone to play with or to just have something that his friends already had, and for me to know that I couldn't give that to him, tore at my heart. The reminders hurt but so did the knowledge that in some small way he was hurting too.

I often just wanted to pull him close and whisper: "I know son, I know."

Every one a blessing

During the months that I was trying for another child and taking the Clomid, my best friend Jo and my brother and sister-in-law both conceived. I should immediately point out that in both instances, I was 100% ecstatic and overjoyed at what was two impending nieces or nephews!

I learnt the hard way through someone very close to me, that being pregnant, indeed giving birth, is no guarantee that you will know the joy of bringing up a child. Conception, pregnancy and birth are all miraculous and the journey to actually give birth to a live, healthy baby is actually a long one, fraught with danger. It's easy to forget just what a miracle it is to get through all three. I really do think that anyone who has experienced the heartache of carrying a child who is then sadly born asleep, or as in my case, felt my own pain at this happening to someone I cared about deeply, you appreciate every single tiny milestone achieved right up until that little baby screams its lungs out in the delivery suite. Having a baby is truly a miracle. Though the most natural thing in the world, it is also too often under-estimated for the amazing miracle it really is.

On 18 October 2010, my darling God-daughter Zara Olive Ann Nightingale came into the world, just 20 minutes after Jo arrived at the hospital. In fact Zara was nearly born on the leather seat of her Daddy's brand new Jaguar car! I was sent a text photo to confirm her safe arrival and literally broke down in tears in the middle of my office. Zara will always know how special she is, I promised her that when I first held her in my arms, but I sincerely hope she will never experience at first hand the reasons why I, and her family, believe she is so special. I love the bones of that little girl and consider her to be my family. I love to hear her say "Auntie Helen". Suffice to say, she is a miracle of life that proves good things eventually happen to good people, some women are meant to be mummies no matter how many hurdles or how much hurt they face on that journey and that despite there being some real rotters, there are some truly wonderful, lovely, generous men in this world.

Six weeks later on 22 November, my brother sobbed down the phone to tell me he was a Daddy. After 4 days hard and stressful labour for my brave sister-in-law Kate, my gorgeous niece, Minnie Joan Makin, finally arrived safely. Kate had an extremely rare complication called Bandl's Ring and we are lucky to have both Kate and Minnie in our lives. I'll never forget the power of love I felt for Zac when he was born, but for Minnie too I felt a really strong love. I immediately felt a bond as her auntie and that as well as Andrew and Kate, I too was responsible for helping nurture this little girl and ensure she knew what a loving family was. It was also bloody weird to think that 'our kid' was now a daddy! He took to it immediately, cried for almost a week and I knew instantly that Kate was a lucky girl to have found him as a daddy for her baby.

The girls, as they turned out to be, had arrived. They were safe, healthy and both absolutely perfect. In the latter stages of both pregnancies their safe arrival had filled my prayers and thoughts. Both Jo and Kate deserved to be mummies, in more ways that I am able to explain. Both would make terrific mummies and both babies were so wanted by their families. My desire to have another child never left me during that time, but definitely, as they got nearer their due dates, my prayers centred around those two babies.

I'd still taken the Clomid, watched my diet, not drunk, cut down caffeine, taken Pregnacare, done my ovulation tests religiously and of course made love in abundance at the right time. I was still focussed and still determined but my prayers centred on those deliveries.

Once Zara arrived, my focus centred on Kate and 'the nut' as Minnie was then known! Once Minnie arrived safely, it was almost like a light switched on.

In recent months, I'd felt greedy praying for myself as well as them. They were already pregnant and I genuinely felt that if there were only so many prayers that could be answered, then those two babies were the priority. I'd felt guilty potentially asking for too much from whoever it was that decided who had babies. Three? You want three healthy babies? One for Jo, one for Kate and then another for yourself? Surely that was asking too much? It didn't mean I wanted one any less and it didn't mean my feelings had changed but it was almost as if I felt that I'd had my chance of being a mum and if that was all it was going to be, so that Jo and Kate's bumps became healthy babies, then thank you, that will do me just fine. As their bumps grew so did my anxiety for their safe deliveries.

The relief when they arrived was certainly because I'd already loved those baby girls for nine months, but I think it was also because now, I could pray for a baby for me. I had room to ask and expect. There was also the additional pressure I immediately piled on myself to provide a playmate close to the girls in age, which I knew was ridiculous but all of a sudden it became important to me. Jo and Zara were as good as blood to me and Minnie was my first blood niece so both were exceptionally special. To be able to have a playmate that could grow as close to them as I was to Jo and Andrew became really important to me.

Overnight, it was OK for me to pray for our baby and with that came a new urgency, a stronger desire and renewed focus.

It was now my time and I was ready.

The IVF chapter was upon me

As the days and weeks went on, the Clomid drugs ran out and my final consultation date got closer. Then the panic really started to set in. I was obsessed with doing everything I could to get pregnant in those last months. I became superstitious, even got slightly OCD such was my paranoia and sensitivity to wanting to be in complete control and to do anything at all that would help me get pregnant.

Looking back it's no wonder those last two months didn't prove fruitful as I put so much pressure on us to conceive within that time, so that we wouldn't need the IVF. The best way to describe how I felt at that time is to liken it to claustrophobia. As time ran out and the window to conceive on our own got smaller, the more and more I felt like I was suffocating, running out of oxygen to breathe. I'm convinced this originated from the fear of showing my last card or taking the last throw of the dice by starting the IVF. As long as I had the IVF option in my locker I still had a chance of a baby. I had an overwhelming fear of having the treatment and it not working and then where would I go and what would I do? Sometimes I really do believe that I didn't feel brave enough to go through with IVF just so that there was still some hope and a chance in the future.

That didn't happen however and as I entered my last month of Clomid I made an appointment to revisit Professor Killick. By the time we went to see him we had past the point of conception for that final month and so there was nothing more we could do. I was spent, I felt spent and I walked into the familiar consultation room already feeling like I'd failed.

My legs felt heavy, my mouth dry and I worried that I wouldn't be able to find the words to tell him it hadn't worked. Strangely we could still have been pregnant at that time, as I hadn't yet had my last period and I kept reminding myself of that as we waited for him to come into the room. I really tried to be positive and confident and believe that this appointment would end up just being a formality. How we'd laugh in a few months at wasting the £95 private consultation fee when all along I was sat there newly pregnant. It was a nice thought, a warming dream but right now, as the Prof finally walked in, it was time to wake up to the reality that we were more than likely not pregnant.

As ever the Prof just made me feel emotional. His warm, kind hearted mannerisms coupled with his wacky humour were the perfect combination to put you at ease, in what he obviously was an expert at knowing, was a very stressful meeting.

He shuffled through the papers in our file, listened to our update about the last 12 months with Clomid, he asked about my general health and my age and all the while I felt like I was waiting for an exam result. It was like he was going through the motions and then any minute now he'd hit us with the result or news he'd known from the start.

One of the Prof's best qualities was his ability to cut to the chase and make decisions very quickly. "Given the relatively quick success with Clomid you had the first time, the fact that you've now been taking it for 12 months and that you are now 37, I think it would be wise to consider IVF."

There it was. We'd been invited into the Last Chance Saloon. In some ways, given the frustrations I'd had and the obvious lack of success, you might perhaps think this news would have been positive. It was a positive next step. It was logical. It was progress. It was however, not something I had really been prepared to hear.

Tears started to roll down my cheeks. I sat there silent, just staring at him for what seemed like minutes but could only have been seconds. I couldn't find any words to say because I just didn't know how I felt about what he'd said. Jason's hand rubbed my leg and he gently squeezed it, which I knew was to reassure me and to say be strong. I could feel my chest tightening as I was obviously struggling to relax and breath slowly. By now I was already starting to fight the huge sobs that were beginning to build up. Jason and Professor Killick were talking, but I have no idea what they were saying. I was at a complete loss as to what to say but I was also at a complete loss as to why I'd suddenly seemingly lost the ability to speak or think.

The problem was really quite simple. Despite the months and months of building up to this moment, I had just realised then and there that I hadn't really allowed myself to prepare for it. I hadn't a clue what it meant to "consider

IVF", what the next step was or what the treatment actually entailed. Here I was now, about to sign up for something that was possibly the biggest event in my life and I hadn't a clue what was going to happen! In fact, those three letters, I.V.F. what the hell were they? What actually was IVF? I was due on in a few days, so what did this mean? Would the treatment start straight away? The questions raced through my mind and I didn't know any of the answers. I was starting to panic and for the second time in that clinic, I broke down and sobbed uncontrollably.

I tried to pull it back, apologising as I always did and desperately tried to compose myself, if for no other reason than we hadn't actually finished the conversation. Professor Killick explained that he would recommend going for the treatment but it was obviously our decision. My mind was racing as fast as my heart, but my thoughts were so unclear I felt that I couldn't possibly make a decision. In reality, the decision of what I had to do right there in that room, had actually been made many months before.

I have always been a huge believer in the power of the mind and that positive thought is an under-rated medicine. I've often thought, particularly with Kate's birthing experience, how lucky we are to be born in a day with all the technological advances and modern medicines that make life more bearable and make the previously impossible actually possible. Modern drugs helped me have Zac so I fully understand and appreciate the power they have had on our lives. On the other hand, I do think that all the drugs and procedures in the world still need a strong mind and a rested soul in order to work effectively. Years ago there was a TV advert where a dad encouraged a young boy by saying "PMA son – Positive Mental Attitude" and it's been a phrase many people of my generation often repeat.

Whilst upset and frustrated, I genuinely did have a PMA throughout the many months of taking Clomid and in order to stay focussed and positive, I had put the thoughts of IVF clear out of my mind. I wouldn't need to know about it, after all, I <u>was</u> going to conceive on Clomid. My positivity had actually put me in a negative situation after all. I hadn't read up on the treatment, spoken to anyone about it and had absolutely no idea what it entailed. I didn't know how long it took, how it happened, who did what…. nothing. Moreover, I had no idea how best to help myself to get the best outcome through the treatment and the thought of it filled me with utter fear and dread. The complete lack of knowledge, of a plan, of any control over the next few weeks of my life was utterly terrifying.

I wasn't ready. I knew I wasn't ready. At best, in everyday life, I am a self-confessed control freak. I was so far out of control in this situation, I didn't even know how best to answer him or talk about it.

"I don't think I can do it yet." I could hear the words coming out in between sobs but it felt like someone else was saying them for me. I mean what was I thinking? Of course I could do it. I had to do it! Here was someone giving me the chance of a child and I was chickening out?! "I don't know anything about it, I've not read anything, I just don't feel ready to go through something so important."

Thankfully, Jason helped me out. "Do we have to start the treatment straight away?" Professor Killick replied that we could have three more months of Clomid if we were happy to do so and schedule the treatment for the end of the third cycle.

It was the signal I needed to get my head back into gear and pull myself together. I must have had an almost physical reaction to the huge relief that washed through me at his words. All of a sudden my thoughts became clearer, my concentration returned and I could again be part of the conversation coherently.

I had felt disappointment, regret and shame in saying I didn't think I could go through with it. I couldn't believe my own ears. This was all I had wanted and been focussed on for so long and here was our opportunity to have a greater chance and I was turning it down. From being a young girl I had always tried to be a brave, determined little fighter that always tried to have a go at anything. If you told me I couldn't achieve something I'd have had a bloody good go to prove that I could. I'd never walked away from a challenge or a fight in my life. Until now.

I remember turning to Jason, almost thankful that the huge tears filling my eyes meant that I could hardly see his face, and I said "sorry." No matter how supportive or involved a partner is through fertility treatment, ultimately the responsibility lies with the one receiving the treatment. There was little more he could do and I felt terrible that in some way I might be letting him down by saying I couldn't go through with it. As ever, Jason was wholly supportive, understanding that as a couple we'd not really looked into what this next stage involved and that obviously I'd not prepared myself.

It was down to me to park the shame and get over that. I had to, there was no time for wasted emotion and energy. It was now down to us both to find out all we could about the treatment and spend the next three months preparing. I had never considered that we would be allowed any more Clomid and so that option hadn't really crossed my mind. Now, the extra three months felt like some sort of reprieve, and I was hugely grateful for it.

I immediately felt lighter, brighter and altogether more positive. Professor Killick gave us a pack of information from the clinic about the IVF treatment and we left with our three additional Clomid cycles feeling we were once more on a positive track.

I started to read the papers he gave us as soon as I got home but I couldn't make head nor tail of them. The IVF journey was described 'easily' in a diagram that I simply couldn't make sense of. The following night I called Jo and asked her a whole load of questions and as she answered I started to fill in the blanks and understand the process a little more.

That night, my period arrived. My disappointment was huge, as ever, but my mood was not as dark as I had thought it might be. I had three more chances now and I was starting to understand the IVF journey. I was stronger, more in control and a whole lot more positive.

The journey starts

Those three months seemed to come and go so quickly. I was learning more about IVF as the weeks went on and slowly began changing my focus from time running out with three more chances to conceive naturally, to time getting closer to a real chance to get pregnant. The shift in psychology was enormous. I didn't try any less in those months but the pain at not being successful was perhaps slightly less that it had been previously. Each time my period arrived it was easier to pick myself up as it helped to think that I was getting closer to the treatment. I also felt less panic at time running out and less desperate to conceive naturally.

I bought a number of books on IVF, PCOS diets and spent evening after evening Googling 'trying for another baby', 'struggling to conceive a second child'. I joined a couple of online chatrooms on websites dedicated to Infertility but was soon too overwhelmed with the jargon and acronyms they used. These girls lived and breathed their situation, they almost seemed to enjoy chatting about their feelings and using these little code words and letters that nobody else could make head nor tail of. I instantly hated it, I didn't get it. I was still me, still spoke English, still dressed the same way, I just wanted to have another child. At that time, I didn't feel part of the infertility world at all, couldn't see that we were all indeed in the same situation and that actually, the lingo and acronyms they used were just because they were all busy in their own lives!

The way I saw my journey panning out at that time was that I was about to do IVF so I was about to have a baby. This really didn't feel like a world I belonged in nor did I want to belong. It hurt too much to see the little angel emoticons or the dates of miscarriages and lost pregnancies. I felt their pain and it really didn't feel good taking on more than I already felt for myself.

Part of the reason I think I also hated the online support sites was also an acute feeling of being an alien in a foreign land. They all seemed to talk about angel babies, struggling seeing couples with a child or children and not being able to bear being around families. I had a child, and my child was alive and often kicking a football by this stage. I had known heartache in trying for my first and my second child, but not to the extent of some of these women. I was also the very person that they found it difficult being around. I read very little that came from someone with children, who was struggling to conceive and so I didn't feel this was the place for me to find the support I needed. Yet I didn't find that support online or in books anywhere else.

We hadn't really told anyone what we were about to embark on the treatment, expect my Mum. This all consuming subject was almost like a hand in front of my face at all times, distracting me, getting in the way of dealing with day to day life. It was like dragging a psychedelic elephant around with you that was huge, heavy and distracting but that nobody else could see. It was something that affected what I thought, how I dealt with things, my concentration, in fact it affected everything every day and yet nobody else could see it and I couldn't talk about it.

Though I was less desperate and panicky I was none-the-less still extremely anxious. My great white knight was about to whisk me off finally from the land of infertility but I had no idea where he was going to take me or if he was actually going to look after me and make me happy after all. Would we have a happily ever after?

There was also the consideration of funding, as there is no funding available in the UK for fertility treatment if either partner already has a child. We had always worked hard and in our early years of marriage we saved really hard too. We both had great jobs for a number of years and with that came two good salaries, plus we had both received redundancy pay outs from previous employers. Our first house had been modest but we had bought it slightly run down and made money doing it up and selling it for our larger family home. Neither of us was in a position of financial support or security from parents or family and that vulnerability and of struggling financially in our younger years, hadn't left either of us. Therefore, all the money we could, we had saved for a rainy day. We weren't rich or well off but we were comfortable and we wanted to be able to provide for our family. What we didn't expect was that we would have to call on our rainy day money to help create our family. But yet, it was indeed a rainy day, in fact it felt like it was pouring down, so we were very fortunate to have savings to call upon.

The consideration that we were choosing to get pregnant to such a degree also weighed heavy on my conscious with regards work and my business partners. I had always been clear when we started the business that Zac was my absolute priority and that in time I wanted to extend the family and try for another baby. Yet now, I felt a small level of apology that I was pro-actively going to need to take time off for maternity leave. The feeling was completely and utterly unfounded and ridiculous as the journey towards pregnancy in terms of a pro-active decision is no different through IVF than it is if you decide to have a baby and have sex on a particular day in your cycle to increase your chances and happen to get caught. Yet for some bizarre reason I felt I was being perhaps deceptive or sly. For some reason the feeling of being obliged to talk about it with them was growing week by week.

The pressure as ever can only last so long. We were having a particularly stressful week and the design studio, headed up by Dom one of my business partners, was really busy. I was leading a design project for a corporate brochure that had needed amends for the umpteenth time and when I'd briefed the guys Dom had snapped at me in his usual direct, curt way. We always got on brilliantly and his occasional directness was usually amusing and I always knew to either laugh at him or ignore him but on this particular day, his retort was my final straw.

I sat back down at my desk and could feel my eyes prick. He hadn't upset me, he hadn't said anything that offended me. Yet his anger from the tense studio that was directed at me was just a push that tipped me over an already delicate imbalance of emotions and by the time our other partner Emma came in from lunch and asked me if I was OK, I could hardly keep the tears from dripping down my cheeks.

By now, I knew I wasn't crying at Dom's response, or indeed at the fact it had made me cry. I knew I was crying at the realisation that I was going to have to tell them that we would probably need to have IVF. That time had come. I took Emma up on the suggestion of a walk outside and we went and sat on a bench overlooking the estuary just near our office. She started to soothe me about "Dom being Dom" and we know he doesn't mean anything by it and then she started to try to make me laugh. "It's not Dom" I could hear myself saying. With that, following a deep intake of breath and what felt like the longest pause I finally told her I was crying because I had been trying for a baby and it was probable that we would need to undergo IVF.

It felt like a confession! Why? It was my business too, it was my life and maternity leave was common throughout the world! I knew I was really crying because I was confirming that I wanted to expand the family which would mean taking time off, which like any business partner, I didn't expect her to be happy about. I think saying the words "we were going to have to go down the IVF route" out loud to someone, was also an emotional drain on me that caused the tears to flow. It was an admission. An admission to myself as much as to her.

An admission of failure perhaps? Inadequacy? Would she view me any differently? It was no longer an issue confined to our bedroom or the clinic. The secret of our struggle was in the open air now. We couldn't conceive and we would need IVF. We needed treatment. We needed assistance. It felt like what should be so natural suddenly became a condition, a problem, something that needed intervention and that fact weighed heavy.

I took some deep breaths, blew my nose and contemplated how I now felt after telling her the full truth. I certainly started to feel lighter but the pain also felt heavier. The reality of 'needing' IVF suddenly made my soul sink to new depths, my heart cracked and a little piece of me curled up and cowered inside. 'Yes, it's me, I'm one of those people, I'm a statistic, I can't create a child on my own. I need to take time out and drugs to help me.' I'd been upset about telling her I was trying for a baby and hoped I'd need to take maternity leave at some stage but now, hearing my own voice admitting I needed to go down the IVF route brought fresh tears to my eyes and made my teeth clench tightly. It was a new feeling of admission of my failings, an acknowledgement I had tried to avoid and done my best to overcome. It was a shame, an embarrassment and a huge anger that I should be in this situation.

Emma was really supportive and we both laughed when she said she certainly hadn't expected that! After a long chat, we returned to the office where we met Dom in the boardroom and I told him the same story. He too was instantly understanding and supportive. In a way it felt like it was enough support from them just for not blowing their tops at me wanting maternity leave, because in having no comprehension of how I was feeling, any other words were just superlatives and of little comfort really. I left the office that evening feeling that another hurdle had been jumped and that we were one step closer to the IVF treatment becoming a reality.

The time passing and learning more about what the next step with IVF might involve made me relax more than I had in the past and got me in a more positive frame of mind for whatever might happen next.

Of course we still took the opportunity that those three months gave us seriously. We desperately would have loved for it to have worked and to have conceived naturally but having the chance to get our heads round the fact that it probably wouldn't, and get used to the idea that we were really already starting the next chapter, seemed to shift our focus from despair at the Clomid not working, to a new found positive focus for the IVF procedure.

Three months and three periods later the next chapter really was about to start.

We had received our appointment for the group introductory session already from our last meeting with Professor Killick. This was a monthly session with all the new couples starting treatment together, listening to a presentation from the entire team, learning more about the process and technical sides of the procedures, meeting everyone involved and a chance to ask questions.

It was also a chance that you might see someone you knew! Jason and I have always been a pretty private couple and this was a subject that we'd not really spoken about much to anyone. Plus, anyone we had spoken about it to, would have been close friends and family and the thought that we might bump into a colleague, client or some other random acquaintance was a total turn off for us both. When we were first told about the meeting we were both dead against going. We'd paid to go private with our treatment and we wanted it to stay private! Professor Killick had explained that many couples found it useful to hear the answers to questions they had not thought to ask themselves and to also realise that there were other people in the same boat. He also explained that to go through the level of detail the team needed to on an individual basis would take up too much of the clinic's time. We understood all that, but still with some trepidation about the whole 'all in it together' scenario, we said we'd see how we felt nearer the time. After a chat about it at home, we felt the need for information was far greater than our fear of being seen so we arranged to attend.

All the uncertainty about whether to go to the session, my usual busy work/home schedule and probably a bit of fear at starting, all meant that I hadn't really considered the obvious practical consideration of us going to the meeting. What would we do with Zac?

Obviously we couldn't take him to the clinic, I'd left it too late for my Mum to come and stay and she lived too far away to come across for a couple of hours. We had a couple of friends we could possibly ask to look after him but then we'd have to tell them what we were doing and I just didn't feel ready to open that can of worms. It would seem odd to just randomly drop Zac off from 6.30pm without saying why. It was something we'd never done before and to anyone who knew us, it would seem really bizarre, especially without an explanation. In the end we asked our neighbours, Giselle's parents, if he could come across, with his pyjamas if needed and we'd pick him up as quickly as we could. I told Sara we were going to see a consultant about trying again and she wished me all the best as she scooped up my baby boy that evening, who was already happy to go and play with his friends.

It was strange to be worrying about our baby boy when we were going off to the clinic. It was also strange to be telling friends what we were doing but it wouldn't have felt right entrusting someone with the care of our baby and then lying to them about why. And yet, speaking the words, then actually leaving Zac to go the clinic, was all extremely surreal. It was a mixture of excitement, nerves and fear of what was to come next. Not just at the meeting, but for our family. What would the future hold? We were taking the first steps to find out.

Staring at the face of frightening statistics

We didn't want to be late given how important the meeting was and having just dropped Zac off we were cutting it fine, so Jason dropped me off at the door and went to park the car. As it happened, with only five minutes until the meeting started, I was seemingly the only one in the waiting room.

Here I was again in the same familiar clinic waiting room. The chairs are arranged facing each other in a square configuration, which every time I sat there, without exception, I wondered at the thinking behind that? Surely people in that situation don't want to sit looking at other people? Seemingly to alleviate the issue of everyone looking at each other, they had placed some huge fake iris plants in the centre of the square and a couple of coffee tables with magazines and leaflets. It is a surreal set up but one that becomes strangely comforting each time you return.

It was strange to be sat there again in that waiting room and yet now be worrying about Zac. We had a child now! Many times I'd sat in those chairs longing for a family, wondering if I would ever have a baby and now here I was again, but unbelievably worrying about my baby, who was being looked after by neighbours! Aside from the worry at whether he was OK, it was a warm, satisfying feeling and I was once again thankful to the team here.

More and more couples arrived, all with the same polite nervous smiles, and the waiting room started to fill up. Usually you only see one or two other couples at most during appointments and quite often you're the only people in the waiting room. To have the room almost full of people was a bizarre experience, everyone discreetly checking everyone else out whilst still trying to avoid eye contact and mind their own business.

I was suddenly conscious that I was on my own. What if they thought I was a single mother, a surrogate or a lesbian? For a fleeting second I was alarmed at what they might think but common sense soon flooded back. What if they did? What did it matter? I could have been any one of those but it didn't matter and wasn't important. In fact I could have been all three, who cares? This clinic was hopefully a saviour for everyone and anyone, whatever their circumstance or preference and I couldn't even believe that those thoughts had entered my head?

I looked around, I didn't know anyone but I suddenly felt a connection. We all wanted something and for a variety of different reasons were all struggling to get it. All walks of life, all ages, all sexes, some same sexes, various sizes, just everyday people but all with a different story. Every couple had a different path that had led us all here to this room on this night. We were all now here together, stood in the last chance saloon, hopeful of a positive outcome. All with the same desires, same rights, same love to share but probably all with different futures and outcomes.

As we were called through to the meeting room, Jason arrived just in time and we walked through the doors together holding hands. I was happy and proud to walk through with Jason. It wasn't anything to do with what anyone else thought of me or of us, it was simply that my buddy, my support, my partner through all of this was here with me, side by side and we were embarking on this together. I remember squeezing his arm as I held him close and we walked into the meeting room. I wasn't first to arrive after all, another twenty or so couples were already seated and we were the last group to arrive.

With a swift glance, I realised I didn't know anyone. If I'm honest it was a relief, though by the time I got seated it was clear that there were some things that were just not important now, and knowing someone in that room was one of them.

Professor Killick had been right, it was useful to be there, to learn more, hear other questions we'd not considered but overall, to realise that there wasn't just Jason and I struggling to have a child, there were many other couples who were in pain too. It was amazing to think that right at the same time we were starting on our journey, there were about 30 other couples starting too! 30! We were both shocked that there would be 29 other couples starting their treatment that same month with us.

The reality of what that actually meant didn't escape me either. Hull's IVF clinic at the time had a tremendous record and was currently the leading clinic in Europe with its success rates at 45%. Still the generally accepted statistic for the IVF success rate is one in three. Was that one in three attempts or one in three couples? Either way there was every chance that a good few of these couples wouldn't ever have a baby.

That stark statistic, that horrifyingly upsetting fact was unshakable from my mind as I sat in that room. It was gnawing away at me that not everyone sat there would have a baby. Not everyone would know the joy of being parents. The stats suddenly became real when you saw the whites of people's eyes. I felt a renewed grief at the situation.

We were sat three quarters of the way back in the room and I couldn't stop staring across the room at all the other couples. It was heartbreaking to know all these couples were feeling as we were feeling and yet, the statistics dictated that some would never know the feeling we had once felt when our newborn baby was handed to us.

Beyond the sadness and anger at the unfairness of it all, I felt like a cheat. I felt like I shouldn't be there, that I didn't belong. Many more of those couples could have already been parents, with the same or previous partners, but I suddenly felt like the odd one out. The greedy one who had come back for more and whose very presence was reducing the chances of others in that room. If Jason and I left the room, would everyone else have a greater chance? If I took up one of the lucky chances of conceiving, would it mean that someone else wouldn't?

I had a child. I had been lucky once. I was a mother and I had been given everything I had prayed for. That night I had kissed my son's sweet head as I left him with friends and promised to tuck him into bed with more kisses and cuddles. I loved bedtime and I loved my precious boy. Now, here I was saying "more please". Whilst others still had yet to realise their dream of being a parent and have their prayers answered, I was wanting more. Not five minutes ago I had been worrying in the waiting room about my child, and now here I was taking the up the space of the few fortunate ones from this group of 30, who were going to conceive. Did one in three mean ten for every thirty? Did that mean that twenty couples, forty people in this room would not have a child?

The sadness, guilt, anger was all consuming. I didn't know these people, in truth I didn't want to get to know them, but I did want them all to be successful. To get to the position of bringing themselves along to this meeting, they would have had to have experienced some level of disappointment or heartache for an extended period of time and to now have a real strength and determination to go through with the treatment. For that alone, I felt they deserved to conceive. But that was not what was to happen, short of a lottery-winning portion of incredible good fortune, disappointment was destined for some. My heart started to beat fast and my mouth went strangely dry. I started to pant and knew I had to try to get a grip of myself and stay focussed on this evening and the meeting ahead. I just had to concentrate on our situation. I could not cry, I must not cry. We were here now, I couldn't walk out and reconsider the treatment simply because I was sorry for the other people there.

I had to bring myself round by considering that perhaps there were reasons already known to some of them that would mean they knew the probability of IVF working was a long shot. I also had to consider that as far as I knew, perhaps some of them too already had children. Perhaps I wasn't the only one.

As the presentation began my concentration shifted and focussed on the team and what they had to tell us. I was amazed that everyone from the consultants to the receptionists, from the nurses to the embryologists all had their turn in explaining what they did and what happened during the treatment. They all had colour coded uniforms and were overwhelmingly passionate and proud about what they did. Just as I had fallen in love with Professor Killick all those years before for the amazing work he did, I felt huge admiration and love for his team, who clearly loved the work they did and were hugely proud of their success.

My thoughts began to centre once more on my family, my body and my chances of conceiving again. I began to concentrate on what Jason and I needed to get through this process. This was me now. In our small family, I was still special, this baby would be special. Forget statistics. Forget the fact that these meetings happen every day all over the UK and the world. We weren't talking 30 people, we were talking hundreds of thousands of people who need assistance in conceiving. From that moment, nobody else mattered, statistics didn't concern me and I had to focus on our family. This wasn't just another cycle, this was my cycle, my next chance to have another child, extend our family and provide a much wanted sibling for Zac. It wasn't that I didn't care about those other couples still or stopped wanting the very best for them, it was just sometimes, there is only so much emotion you can deal with and at that moment I realised mine would be best spent focussing on my own situation.

I had prepared questions that I wanted answering and as the presentation went on I chipped in with the occasional question. At the end, they invited questions and I waded through my list. By the end of the session I'd probably asked 8 of the 10 questions! I didn't care what anyone thought, in fact I couldn't understand why more people didn't ask more. It was as if they'd had received some secret information booklet that I'd missed out on, or they weren't really bothered about what was to come. Either way, I'd got my answers, some I understood more than others, but overall, it was a useful session and I felt it was worthwhile.

At the end, the senior nurse spoke to us and said that a lot of my questions would be answered as we went through the treatment and that I should try not to worry too much. She obviously thought I was some sort of nutter! This was the first time we met Denise, who would be a huge part of our treatment going forward. We took the opportunity to ask her if we could arrange for Professor Killick to do our transfer of the embryo as he had been our consultant through trying for our first child. She was quick to make it clear that the consultants were extremely busy and didn't always do the treatment. The nurses in the clinic did the transfers almost all of the time and were highly skilled at doing so! That told us! We were both alarmed at not being able to guarantee Prof Killick would be involved and at being told so in no uncertain terms.

I could feel my eyes pricking. It probably wasn't anything to do with the answer to the question. I didn't care if Boy George put the embryo back as long as I conceived. It was probably more to do with it being the end of the meeting and me needing to release all the pent up stress that had obviously been building.

She softened then and explained that it was normal to feel anxious but that the whole team were there to help see us through it and the best thing I could do was relax.

Denise, we would soon learn, was the head of the unit and a critical member of the team. The consultants floated in and out but Denise ran the clinic. Her apparent hardness and abrupt style were to prove to be a Godsend to me in later months and I would grow to love her immensely but at this moment, when I first encountered her, I just wanted to get out of the clinic, get home and have a bloody good cry!

We walked into Sara's where Zac was sat in his pyjamas quite happily watching a film with the girls. He was happy to see us but had had a lovely time and wasn't that keen on coming home! It was lovely to hold him and we had extra cuddles before bed that evening.

It's all in the preparation

Two days after the group meeting I called the clinic to tell them I had started my period. I was told to start taking the pill and that by the end of the week I'd be sent a letter with my next consultant dates and our first invoice. I needed to pay the invoice before they would release the drugs but they looked forward to seeing us in the next few weeks.

The letter arrived with dates and the invoice. It was really the first time I had looked at the true financial cost of the treatment but surprisingly, given the four figure number at the bottom of the bill total, I was strangely calm. It was a serious amount of money and I had always thought that when it came to seeing the invoice or writing out the cheque I would probably panic or even pass out! Now, as I hurriedly wrote the cheque to get it back to the clinic as quick as I could so that they would release my drugs, it was one of the easiest things in the world. I could buy eight pairs of Laboutins with the money I was spending but honestly, writing a cheque for that amount for shoes would be a lot more painful! Money was suddenly not important. If that's what it cost, that's what it cost and there was no point worrying now. We were fortunate to have the money at that moment in time and we didn't think twice about spending it on the treatment.

We were also about to spend a whole lot more money that hurt a lot more! I had got it into my head that our lives were about to hugely change and we needed to enjoy our time as just the three of us as much as we possibly could. We were also aware that if we were going to get pregnant, and then have a newborn, it may be some time before we would be able to get away and so to enjoy time together and help me relax, we decided to book a holiday.

To this day I still can't understand my thinking in those weeks before we went away. All I could think about was how important it was that I relax.

Looking back now, I can see that in trying to stay calm, all I was doing was stressing myself out further, unnecessarily so, but in those weeks, there was no telling me or indeed I was beyond understanding that this was what was happening.

Even choosing where to go on holiday proved to be stressful. I almost became panicked at making the wrong decision and choosing a holiday that wasn't relaxing. For a number of years we'd had great holidays in villas we'd rented in Portugal and Cyprus but for some reason I felt that doing our own catering and entertaining Zac on our own 24/7 wouldn't be relaxing enough for me. I decided that a hotel would be our best bet this time, having someone else to cook and clean for us, to make our beds and to have children around for Zac to play with.

Choosing a hotel proved to be a nightmare. Probably every other one we looked at would have been perfectly fine but none at the time were what I was looking for. The problem was, I didn't know what I was looking for, other than something that would be 'relaxing'! I wanted Zac to have a great time and play with other children so we thought a kids club was a good idea. Relaxation was a priority so I thought a nice spa was a must and then of course we wanted a nice room, great food, the needs list when on and on.

With work commitments and impending treatment dates we were pretty limited on when we could go. We started looking on the Saturday night and were to fly out the weekend after. I was searching for a four/five star family friendly hotel and the Internet was throwing hundreds of options. We realised that we were now in fact actually looking at the most expensive single week to go away in the entire year, the last week of the school summer holidays with a return flight on the bank holiday weekend!

The more 'family friendly' a hotel appeared to be, the more I thought I would hate it, because it would be full of over-friendly families that I really didn't want to be on holiday with. The more activities or facilities they seemed to have for kids, the less attention they seemed to spend on nice furnishings, food or facilities such as a gym or spa for Jason and I. And now, because of the week we had to go away, we were spending more money than we had planned, the total was going up by the day and this put more pressure on ensuring we chose a great holiday. I was now really worried that I'd spend all this money and end up choosing something we all hated! I was looking for a relaxing 'dream' holiday that was so full of contradictions it didn't really exist!

After several days of indecision, by the Wednesday the flights had gone up £300!

It all sounds utterly ridiculous now, a complete waste of energy but that is just a tiny example of how the anxiety was starting to engulf every area of my life. Worry after worry after worry and often worrying about what I would worry about next. Even booking a fabulous holiday in the sun was too much to cope with at that moment.

In the end we chose a five star hotel in Paphos, Cyprus that was listed in a Times newspaper article that I found online as one of the top ten family friendly hotels. Described as a luxury, five star family beach hotel the website boasted: "a comfortable combination of modern design elements, sleek facilities and family-friendly features: because having children doesn't mean that you have to sacrifice good taste...". It looked and sounded perfect but of course cost a fortune. It was ridiculous!

We got to the stage where we thought 'what the hell!'. It would be our last holiday with just the three of us, we'd never been to a hotel like this before and after all we had just 2 days before we were to due to fly out so we needed to decide quickly! Bugger it, we quickly paid, packed and set off.

As soon as we arrived, the hotel took our breath away and we were thrilled with our choice. That night however, our hearts sank, as it appeared our room was situated close to a noisy road and next to a constant banging corridor door. We both felt like crying. Ordinarily we might be annoyed at such a problem, we'd look at it in perspective for what it was, just an unsatisfactory room and sort it out levelheaded the next morning. That night it felt like the end of the world, like everything was up against us. It was just another example of how the strain of the treatment made anything else that was negative always feel like the final straw. The smallest complication exploded into a catastrophic problem.

That said, a 3am call to reception then a complaint to the manager at breakfast the next morning and we were swiftly moved to a fabulous room at the other end of the hotel overlooking the sea.

The rest of the holiday was a dream. Beautiful room, amazing food and a wholly lovely experience. Every detail was super special and it was beyond what we were hoping and looking for. Once there however, we didn't put Zac in kids club at all and I didn't visit the spa once. We were having such a lovely time as a family together, just the three of us that we didn't feel the need or desire to spend any time apart. Zac made friends round the pool and was happiest pottering in and out, playing with his toys by the side of the sun beds or doing his favourite past time of people watching, or rather staring!

The other holiday makers were friendly but not overly so, and when Roger Black and his family turned up half way through the week, a few of us all winked and had a bit of a gossip at the new resident celebrity, and it was lovely to be sociable without being in each others space too much.

One of the other mums I got chatting to had three very small children with the eldest seeming to be only just a little older than Zac, who was by now just three and a half. She turned out to be a private maternity nurse from London, who had had all three children through IVF and had wasted no time in having the next one each time she fell pregnant.

She was the first stranger I spoke to about my treatment. It was a revelation just how telling someone that I was about to start the treatment felt really liberating. We were sharing stories and I was listening to her experiences picking up hints and tips and all the time feeling lighter, freer and less like a freak! She made me feel excited about the prospect and made me feel hopeful.

It reminded me of leaving NCT (National Childbirth Trust) classes just before I had Zac when we were told that as women we were built to have children and we were made especially to give birth. I left that class feeling so empowered and wanting to shout, "I am a woman!" She made me feel like that again and for the first time I really felt positive. Her career had meant she had witnessed many births and new mums so her advice was very down to earth and not at all like any textbooks. She made light of how many embryos to put back and even said she had told her consultant to stick an extra one in for good measure and so the last time she had three put back without her husband knowing! Each time however she delivered one healthy baby. She was very relaxed about the whole experience but then with three beautiful babies and a loving, obviously patient husband, it was no surprise!

I walked back to Jason on our sun beds smiling, not knowing how on earth I was going to explain why I felt so excited. I was just supposed to have gone to fetch fresh towels!

That night, Zac, who was by now obsessed with chicken kebabs, had requested that he have his dinner by the pool, which meant he would eat about 5pm. Jason and I planned to get changed ready for dinner after he ate, then we'd all go to the sushi restaurant later that evening, armed with colouring books to occupy Zac while we ate our dinner.

As Zac tucked into his kebab, Jason offered me a gin and tonic, which sounded perfect. In preparation for the treatment, I hadn't had a drink in months but in the warmth of the evening sun, my favourite time of the day, I really fancied a tall G&T. It was gorgeous…but went straight to my head. After just one drink I was totally pissed! I stumbled back to the room, struggled to get dressed and ended up throwing my hairbrush across the room in temper, which is something I'd never ever do normally! I needed to lean on the buggy to help me walk through the reception, tripped over the kerb on the street outside and as I finally sat down in the restaurant, the lights on the trees outside seemed to be spinning round and round in front of me. I was absolutely sozzled and all Jason could do was laugh at me! This was one of the more fun side effects of preparation for the treatment and one Jason still hasn't let me forget!

As it was, the rest of the holiday was fabulous and we all had a terrific time.

We're on!

Three weeks after we landed back, we had our first appointment and as we sat in the familiar waiting room again, for the first time in recent months I felt a flush of anxious excitement.

The process was explained, we went through a dozen forms giving various consents and we were handed a huge paper carrier bag of drugs. In some small way I felt a bit better about handing over so much money when I saw the huge amount of drugs we were being given but in another way, it filled me with horror at the thought that all those drugs were going to all end up inside me over the next few weeks.

Our nurse Dawn very carefully explained each step to us and I tried desperately to take it all in. I occasionally asked her to go over certain points again and finally, slowly, for each stage, the pennies started to drop and I knew what we had to do.

The clinic only ever spoke about the very next stage in front of you and would never talk about what would happen after that, preferring to placate anxious questions with "we'll talk about that at your next appointment" or "don't worry about that for now, concentrate on the next week ahead". For me, a control freak and constant planner, it would prove frustrating over coming months as I always felt better knowing what was coming and when, but that day sat in the small consulting room, it was reassuring that all I had to take in was the very next step and learn how to inject myself. My mind was racing and my brain bursting so the little bit of detail given was appreciated that afternoon.

This stage would last for 4 weeks and I had to inject myself in the stomach every day. I'd known it was coming having spoken to Jo and read all about it in my books. As someone who can pass out at the sight of needles or blood and who has a zero pain threshold, the prospect of the injections wasn't something I'd been relishing. But, like with most elements of pregnancy, childbirth and motherhood, you somehow find that steely grit within you that gets you through the most horrid circumstances that are thrown your way, that previously BK – Before Kids – you would have run from or passed out at.

I wasn't looking forward to the prospect of injecting myself at all but had decided I just had to get on with it and thought that if I took a deep breath, closed my eyes and stuck the needle in quickly, I would be able to cope and everything would be fine.

Oh how wrong could I be? I can laugh now but I honestly thought I would just pick up a needle, close my eyes or look away, take a deep breath, stick it in and pull it out. Job's a good 'un! No, there is no just picking up the needle, certainly no way you can do it with your eyes closed and the serum takes forever to get into your tummy! In fact, breathing is the only part of my fantasy that was accurate!

The intricacies of unwrapping two needles, the syringe, carefully unwrapping the hygienic wipe and wiping the bottle and then putting it all together, all made me feel slightly uneasy even before I had started to think about injecting myself! Our nurse helped and explained that after wiping the bottle you drew the liquid out with a green needle into the syringe, then took that needle off and replaced it with a smaller yellow needle and you were then ready to inject.

With the delicate needles and need to keep it all sterile, then having to carefully draw the correct amount of solution without any air bubbles, there was certainly no way this was going to be a quick procedure each night!

Then it was time to inject. I was shocked that she wanted me to do it there and then in front of her! Here? Now? In this room? It seemed that all of a sudden my actual treatment was really starting. I was suddenly terrified that I hadn't really psyched myself up to stick this bloody thing into myself!

My 'just have to get on with it' attitude kicked in and I took hold of the needle. It had to be done, there was no way it was going to be any easier with Jason doing it for me, in fact that was sure to be a one way track to divorce. I would just have to suck it up and crack on.

I was told to pinch my tummy anywhere below the belly button. This was easy and a flash of disappointment at just how easy it was to grab a sausage of flab across my midriff did cross my mind but was swiftly quashed as my thoughts returned to the needle I was holding in the other hand. "Rest it on your tummy at an angle and then gently push it into your tummy" she said. The words were so easy but the action almost impossible. Holding my 'sausage' I put the needle to my skin but immediately jerked and pulled it away. It bloody hurt! My God, the end of the needle was really sharp and it really, really hurt! And I'd only just put it against my skin! How the hell was I going to push it in if it hurt so much just placing on my tummy?

I tried again, and again and then tried on the other side. My hand was shaking, then my arm started shaking and as much as I was telling myself to push it in, I just couldn't move my wrist forward to do so. It was like an invisible force field that I couldn't penetrate and try as I might, I just couldn't push that needle in.

I can only think that having had that small pain when I first placed the needle on my skin, my mind was then playing tricks and as I knew that pushing it in would hurt, therefore it simply wouldn't allow it. I suppose it's alien to actually, purposefully hurt yourself or indeed do something pro-actively that you know is going to hurt. I kept thinking it wouldn't be too bad if you could inject as I'd previously imagined by just turning away and stabbing it in and out! Yet this minute needle at the end of the syringe would have snapped off for sure if I had done that, plus there was also a syringe full of liquid and I needed to ensure every drop went in. It was clear there would be no rushing this job that was for sure.

More than five minutes passed and it was starting to get embarrassing. Dawn and Jason were lovely, in fact really, really lovely. I started to wonder if Dawn had ever actually tried to do this herself and decided probably not, though she couldn't have been any more encouraging if she had, to be honest. The fact was, there was only one person to move us all forward from this room, and that person was now sniffling at how sorry she was! I started apologising to them both for the amount of time it was taking, then started getting angry with myself for being such a 'wuss' and gave myself a good stern talking to.

Before I knew it, I pushed it in. Actually it was ok, in fact it was so much better than when I first touched my skin with the end of the needle. Holding my sausage with one hand, the other slowly squeezed the top of the syringe releasing the liquid. It seemed to take forever to empty and no matter how hard I pushed it; the liquid would only empty out at its own slow pace. That was something I'd not anticipated either.

Pressing down on my skin, I then slowly pulled the needle out and it was all over! I felt like such big baby but then I also felt tremendous! Jason gave me a huge squeeze and said he was really proud of me and kept saying well done over again. I was actually quite proud of myself as I had been completely taken aback at just how hard the actual physical side of injecting myself had been, compared to the psychological will. The saying 'the mind's willing but the body's weak' perfectly summed it up.

Just another 27 times to go!

Every night we'd try to remember to take the serum out of the fridge a couple of hours before I needed to inject so that it was at room temperature. Overall the injections were fine, not a joy but bearable. The odd time we forgot to take it out of the fridge and as the cold liquid went into my warm tummy it really hurt and then itched like crazy. A couple of times I bruised or the area swelled up and once I think I hit a blood vessel as this huge big black lump ballooned under the skin so I stopped and moved to the other side.

Jason was a rock, helping me remember to do it, preparing all the needles with me and giving words of encouragement the odd times I needed it. If the area was itchy or sore, he'd rub my tummy and tell me how proud he was of me. In his own way he was going through it all with me and I was grateful even just for the fact that he took the time out of whatever he was doing, to sit with me whilst I did it.

I'd read that some husbands or partners do the injections but I think this would have been worse for me. I'm sure I would have lashed out if Jason had done it to me and we both agreed that it would be better for me to get on with it, rather than risk any arguments or violence!

For months now I'd been preparing for the treatment, reading books and surfing the Internet on how best to look after myself to give us the best chance. As the days went on and each injection brought us closer to the transfer of embryos, the intensity of my energies to ensure I was doing everything possible intensified.

I'd not had caffeine for weeks, or alcohol for months. I was eating carefully ensuring I had low GI foods to give me energy, having multi-vitamins with folic acid every day and trying to drink as many fluids as possible.

And yet despite all the healthy living, migraines were an unfortunate side effect of the drugs that made me quite poorly. Twice during those weeks I couldn't make it into the office, as I literally couldn't lift my head from the pillow. They would start as a build up of pressure late in the afternoon and slowly worsen as the day progressed. I'd suffered from headaches in the past but these were more intense and more regular than I'd ever had before. Most days I just felt I had a tight band around my head with just a general fogginess all the time.

Forgetfulness and lack of concentration were two other side effects that I found hard work, especially at work. I was constantly conscious that we were having the treatment because I just didn't feel myself. It was a struggle sometimes to concentrate on the most basic of conversations.

I started acupuncture sessions having read that it was a good alternative compliment to IVF treatment. Randomly there was a Chinese herbal and alternative remedy shop in a shopping centre across the road from my work. I called in to enquire if they could help and had a lovely chat through my situation with a young Chinese girl who was translator to a lovely Chinese man called Han, who turned out to be the doctor. They seemed to think they could help and said they'd assisted with fertility issues previously. They recommended acupuncture and acupressure for a series of weeks ahead of the transfer. I booked a five-week session, got a bit of discount for bulk booking and started my course that day.

Lying in a room just off a shopping centre mall might not seem the most relaxing place to be but as I lay there all alone with nearly 20 needles all over my body, I really felt totally relaxed. I realised that this was probably the first time in years I had had an hour, all on my own, with nothing to do, nothing to think about. It was bliss. If I had a small amount of time on my own on occasion I was always guilt ridden with jobs round the house that needed doing, or my head full of things I needed to get sorted at work. Now, here, the whole purpose was to relax and so I promised myself that I would empty my head of any thoughts and indulge myself for the hour. It really was therapy in itself.

After half an hour chilling out with the needles, Han, returned and started the acupressure. He pressed, rubbed, flicked, stroked and kneaded pressure points all over my face, head and neck. There were certain points, especially from my temple to just above my ear where the pain was excruciating. It was amazing to think I had been walking round with no idea how tender that spot was, even a gentle touch seemed to hurt like hell but the relief was tremendous! Each week I looked forward to the treatment and every time, I didn't want it to end. I slept like a log that night, and the night after too, and I felt calmed by the simple fact that it was worth the expense for just that alone.

And yet, whilst the acupuncture itself was relaxing and making me feel in control of the situation to some degree, leaving work on time to get there and keep my appointments, brought its own degree of stress. Time and again I'd run into the store late for my appointment all hot and bothered which was a constant source of amusement to Han. Why would I spend all this money on relaxing when I would get stressed out trying to get there at all? I'd also arrive more often than not without having had my lunch against Han's recommendations as the needles tended to hurt more if you hadn't eaten. Sometimes I'd grab a bag of crisps from Superdrug round the corner from his shop, hoping I could throw them down me and that it would make some difference. It didn't and only served to make me later for my appointment and then stress about my cheesy Quavers breath as Han lent over me working his magic! Again, why put myself through that stress?

During one appointment, as Han was carefully inserting the needles I could faintly hear the mall music system playing 'All that she wants is another baby'. The irony and what I thought at the time, perhaps the poignancy, didn't escape me and after I got Han to listen, we had a giggle and both crossed our fingers. Han was so gentle and seemingly so understanding despite hardly speaking a word of English, it was nice and calming just to be in his presence. I felt he actually really did care about what he was doing and felt safe and relaxed in his clinic. When I first asked his name, I patted my tummy and said, "If it's a boy!" and we both laughed. It was nice to be with someone whom I could be honest with about my situation and whom I felt really wanted it to work out well as much as I did.

Whilst I was focussed on the start of the treatment, Zac of course was continuing to surprise us with new expressions and interests that showed he was growing up fast. Jason and I would often ask each other how he knew something or where he got an expression or fact. It seemed every time we looked back at a photograph on our phones, even from just a few weeks ago, we could see how much he had changed each time. It was alarming.

For months I'd put off redecorating one of the spare rooms and moving Zac out of the nursery. He was nearly four now and was sleeping and playing in a soft, cream nursery room with a huge teddy bear mural on one wall. He hadn't said anything about it but I knew his friends that came to play all had 'big boy rooms' with dinosaurs, pirates or Cars 2 and that he really should be moving on with his own newly decorated room. He deserved it. After all, it wasn't his fault that we'd kept him in the nursery because the thought of moving him out and having an empty nursery, just waiting to be occupied, had previously felt too much to bear.

I now started to think about his new room and began to get excited. He was obsessed with pirates and I found a gorgeous pirate themed room that was stylish but playful at the same time. I started to make plans for his room and I allowed myself to be giddy about getting the nursery back to being a true nursery, which was a warm, lovely feeling.

Telling the world

Injection by injection I felt I was getting a step closer to having a baby. I really felt more and more excited about the prospect and my mind was full every day of baby names, working out dates I'd be due and so it went on. I felt wholly positive about the expected outcome and really felt that I was on a journey heading towards being a mum again. I was really excited, almost like the feeling when you know you're pregnant before the 12 week scan and you're dying to tell everyone though you know you shouldn't just yet.

During the time we were having difficulty conceiving Zac and were taking the fertility drugs I felt embarrassed, ashamed, and concerned people would think I was a failure. I didn't want to tell anyone and really felt it was a dirty big secret. This time I was more open in talking to friends and in fact, found it a huge support. Close friends rallied round asking for updates on progress and keeping my spirits high. I met girlfriends for lunch and they'd ask about every detail and I felt excited, giddy and a strange sense of pride at my impending motherhood.

Given the odds, my positivity was strange to some degree but I felt that as I'd had a successful pregnancy before and no obvious reason for not conceiving, I was confident that I would be one of the positive statistics. Every day, every injection, every acupuncture appointment and every time I turned down a coffee or gin and tonic, I was getting a step closer and I couldn't wait.

It was around this time that we celebrated our company's birthday and, as had become tradition, myself and Emma took ourselves off for a pamper day to commemorate what we saw as a huge achievement. We were still in business and doing well and we liked to take time out to pat ourselves on the back. Emma chose a heated wrap treatment but having filled in their wellbeing form on arrival and detailed the drugs I was currently taking, I was advised against choosing the wrap for myself and was recommended a session of Reiki. Now I'm never really sure what I believe when it comes to alternative treatments but I do believe that if something relaxes you and doesn't in fact stop you from conceiving, then it can only be a good thing. As I lay on the warm towelling mattress I could sense the therapist's gentle hands working their way up my body, stopping to hover over different areas from my toes all the way up to my head. I really had to stop myself from laughing at times as I could sense her flicking the air above me. Despite struggling to compose myself and not giggle, I could actually see the value of just lying in the peaceful half-light with nothing else to do but relax in the moment for sixty minutes. And so, I tried to forget what the therapist must have looked like over me and put the experience down to a thoroughly enjoyable relaxation session.

That was until she reached my face. My eyes were closed tight but I could sense the warmth of her hands over my mouth. All of a sudden painful thoughts about why we were doing the IVF treatment came flooding into my head. All the hurt of all those negative tests were suddenly at the front of my mind and a deep fear of perhaps never succeeding sent shivers right through my body. Within seconds I felt freezing cold despite the warmth of the electric blanket beneath me. I could feel my throat constricting and I kept swallowing trying to relieve the discomfort. My eyes were starting to itch and I could feel the familiar water building up as tears began to form and then slowly fall down my cheeks. I sniffed to shake off the sobs. I tried to clear my throat, swallow, sniff again but all the time her hands were above my face so I was unable to fully give my head a shake to fight off the obvious tears that were by now falling so fast they were running straight into my ears.

It was then that my throat made a sobbing sound and I had to clear my throat and apologise. "I'm sorry, I'm not sure why I'm crying, it just suddenly happened." By now I was crying my eyes out, I couldn't stop the tears, couldn't control the sobs and it had taken me completely by surprise.

The therapist stepped back and tried soothing me. She didn't seem surprised or fazed at all. "You have something that you are really concerned about, something that is filling your thoughts but you aren't talking about it, you're keeping it all to yourself. This tells me you need to let it out. You need to talk more. You need to let go, let people in and stop holding all that hurt and worry inside." At her words I gasped a huge sob, as I knew exactly what she was referring to. She had no idea, but I knew she had hit the nail on the head. She was right. I had so much going on inside my heart and my head that even I was astounded at how much of a burden it was becoming. I will never know if the timing was coincidental or whether indeed, the Reiki therapy did in fact seek and find where I needed tension releasing, but I do know that the session had a profound impact on my life that day and I realised I needed to stop bottling up my fears and emotions. It frightened me. The power of emotion and my body's reaction had alarmed me that afternoon and I knew then I would have to be very careful moving forward on what was obviously going to be an increasingly stressful and emotional journey.

The thought of the treatment was mostly all consuming. It impacted every single thought or action, every single day. From the food I ate, what I drank, my ability to concentrate, right through to whether my little boy had a pirate bedroom or not! It affected when we went on holiday and what sort of holiday. It impacted what time I had to leave meetings to get to acupuncture and so it went on and on. There was hardly a minute I didn't think about it or had to consider it.

Sometimes I'd wonder if people could tell just by looking at me. I had this huge thing going on in my life and yet most people around me had no idea. Often I would just want to scream: "Do you know what we're going through?", "Have you any idea how messed up I'm feeling right now?" To have this huge distraction in my life was both deeply painful and extremely exciting, but having to keep it to myself was a strange and restricting feeling. I'm a natural talker and have always worn my heart on my sleeve, so to keep what felt like a huge secret to myself was often alien to me. I remember a similar feeling when my beloved Granma died and I was in such pain on the inside when everyone else was carrying on with day to day life, that I just wanted to scream in the street "Hey, I've just lost my Granma guys, my heart is literally breaking over here!"

I found myself starting to talk about it more. I'd sometimes hear myself telling somebody what we were doing and even surprise myself at hearing the words. At the time I just wanted to tell the world. I felt so sure that I was on my way to having a baby and for the first time in a long time I just felt so excited. At other times I just felt so shockingly poorly and either dopey or agitated that it was almost a relief to share with people what I was doing, in that I almost got a sense of support simply by explaining what was going. It was like a defence or excuse almost. I was well on in the journey and my excitement was building day by day.

I visited the clinic where a scan confirmed I had successfully down regulated. This basically meant they had closed down my body's natural processes so that, through the drugs, they could control the production of eggs and thickening of the womb lining, as they required. Injections in my leg then started and if I thought the tummy ones were bad, it was much worse in my leg! These were slower to go in and a lot more painful as there was more muscle than fat. The tops of my legs bruised really badly that week but I was told this was to be expected and so worried a little less.

On the Wednesday I had my first scan to see if the follicles, in which the eggs grow, were growing. The nurses were pleased to see that I had a good number of follicles and they were indeed growing well. I had another positive scan on the Friday, which was just one week before my planned appointment for the eventual harvest, or retrieval of the eggs. Just one week to go!

The IVF clinic was at the Women and Children's Hospital in Hull and I was fortunate to work just 10 minutes away in the car. I'd book the appointments out in my diary and rush to the scans and get back as quickly as I could. That Friday I walked back into the office, straight into a meeting, feeling 10 feet tall. Emma had by now learnt not to ask how I was, but this time looked my way across the desk as I gathered my papers for my next meeting and just said "All alright?". "Yes" I said with a huge grin. "Looks like we're on for next week!"

It's not all plain sailing

That weekend I had horrendous tummy ache. It was a cross between period pain and a stomach bug cramp. I didn't know what was wrong with me and where to put myself, as I had no other symptoms. I just felt really rough and didn't feel like doing anything. Later on Saturday evening I felt a wave of morning sickness. It felt really weird to have that familiar feeling again and even stranger knowing I couldn't possibly be pregnant!

A twinge of a headache that night progressed to a full on migraine when I woke on Sunday morning and my morning sickness got progressively worse. I felt on the brink of throwing up constantly and strong odours made my stomach turn instantly. I felt tired and began to question what on earth I was thinking in trying to get pregnant when I knew how sick I'd felt carrying Zac. What was I doing? By Monday morning I woke up with a sore throat as well and I felt absolutely rotten. Yet I got up and thought nothing more of it other than it must be some reaction to the drugs and the start of a common cold.

I gave Zac a squeeze and felt the warmth of his 'just off the pillow' hair on my cheek and my tummy flipped with love for him. I loved that first cuddle in the morning when he just wanted to curl up in your arms and close his eyes once more. The nausea rose again and I was gutted to have to end our cuddle and quickly stand up straight. He looked alarmed but soon shrugged and went to investigate where his Cheerios were.

I went to my next scan appointment later that day and explained to Denise that I was feeling really poorly and had had a bad weekend. I told her about the headaches, the tummy pains and the nausea. She scanned me and after a few minutes looking at both my ovaries on the screen she confirmed that I had over stimulated and had symptoms of OHSS (Ovary Hyper Stimulation Syndrome). Over the weekend my body had massively reacted to the stimulation drugs and my ovaries were now huge and bursting with oversized follicles. "No wonder you have tummy ache!" she said.

Though comforted that there was a reason why I had felt poorly, I had noticed that Denise sounded somewhat concerned. She took me into one of the consultation rooms and explained the situation. This was not an uncommon side effect but one that they take seriously and one that could make you extremely poorly. I was alarmed to learn that if my ovaries couldn't be slowed down, or de-stimulated I could be hospitalised.

She explained that we needed to get my ovaries to slow down and the only way to do that was to stop the injections immediately and 'coast' for the remainder of the week. There was a chance that if they didn't slow down during coasting, and we proceeded, that any baby conceived would be fine with all those hormones flying round, but I would be extremely poorly. It was then that she told me there was a real chance we might have to cancel this cycle and start again.

I had only popped out of the office for a routine scan! I felt like a bus had hit me. Cancelling this treatment was not an option for me. That was not part of any plan I had in mind! I was having IVF and I was going to have a baby in nine months! I honestly had a single-track vision of what was going to happen and that single track was positive, productive but now seemingly somewhat naïve and unrealistic. It was a massive shock and a huge blow. I was completely unprepared for anything like this.

I was torn between listening to her advice and wanting to do the right thing but also desperately doing whatever it took to continue with this cycle. Of course I didn't want to end up in hospital and given how poorly I felt, I actually knew deep down that this could be a real possibility, but the thought of not continuing and cancelling the cycle was terrifying. I just couldn't believe what I was hearing.

There was nothing I could do. I could hear myself almost pleading with Denise not to cancel. We were sat on low chairs, looking at each other and I was wringing a soggy tissue in my hands. I knew I was sniffling but I was trying so hard to sound in control. My head was banging, throat tightening and sitting on the low chairs was killing my swollen stomach as I bent forward towards Denise trying my best to look 'not so stimulated' in the hope that doing so would help convince her to proceed.

"Please, please don't cancel I was crying inside." Please just try to see if my levels come down. She said that if I fully understood the risks and was willing to proceed we would agree to 'coast' and see if the levels dropped significantly by Wednesday. A huge rush of relief literally washed over me. Her words at that moment had such a monumental impact I'm surprised I literally didn't collapse back into the chair. It felt like some sort of reprieve. I still had a chance. I might be poorly but at least we could have a go and I felt like I had been given a gift! That's all I wanted was the chance. I could put up with feeling this way for a couple more days if that is what it took and I remain immensely grateful to Denise for giving us the opportunity that day. I'm still not sure what cancelling would have done to me but I know it would have crushed a bit of my spirit and positivity that may never have returned. I would never have put my life at risk as Zac was always my priority and he needed his Mummy, so proceeding at all cost was not an option. Yet to push myself to the nearest limit, to give it my absolute all within reason was my only way to approach the treatment in the first place. To be told you have to cancel because of how your body reacts, I am sure must be crushing for any woman. Fortunately this was not the case for me this time.

After being told my sore throat was not related and was just a sore throat, I called in at the pharmacy before I left the hospital, bought some Locket lozenges and called Jason. How on earth would I even start to tell him this latest news? He too would freak at the thought of possibly cancelling the treatment.

The most frustrating thing for me was that there was nothing at all that I could do to change the situation. I just had to remain positive. I eventually made it back to the office though I had no idea how I was going to just sit back down at my desk and pick up my work where I'd left off. Mentally I was drained, emotionally I was spent and physically I was by now undeniably in agony, probably with the visual image of how swollen my insides were with my massive bloated belly.

As it was, I couldn't just sit down and pick up my work. As soon as I looked at Emma and she looked at me to see that everything was OK, I just broke down. My head was pounding, I felt so sick and now my throat was tightening by the minute too. I was still in shock. Cancel my treatment? Be hospitalised? It was the last thing I was expecting and it was almost too much to bear.

We have lift off!

Despite being told that there was nothing I could do to slow the stimulation or reduce the symptoms I spent the next few days trying to remain calm and relaxed. It was something to focus on even if it didn't make any actual physical difference it was definitely helpful in focussing the mind.

I had a strange euphoric feeling inside. I just wanted to shout out "I'm going to have a baby", so much so I found myself telling people, acquaintances, and clients, even complete strangers that I was going through IVF. Almost as the words came out of my mouth I couldn't believe what I was saying. "Shut up Helen!" I'd say to myself. What on earth was I thinking? But I simply couldn't help it. I was beyond giddy. I was so excited that in just nine months time I'd have my longed for baby and I wanted as many people as possible to help share my joy as early as possible. Most people wished me well and seemed pleased for us and I naturally took this as them sharing my joy that I would soon become a mummy again. Each time I had a conversation like that, it felt like we were already celebrating the fact that I was lucky enough to have the treatment, to have a chance of pregnancy and that I was about to have another baby. In my darker moments I realised this was utterly ridiculous and I was obviously getting carried away. This frenzy was frightening but it was something I struggled to curtail.

This was it! It was like we'd been rehearsing for ages and the main event was going to start this week. We really were on the first rung of that very exciting ladder and despite the worry and pain; I was so very excited and couldn't wait to get cracking.

On the other hand, I was also terrified, which was equally as strange a feeling to be having. This was it indeed. A game changer. Life as we knew it was effectively ending and there was no turning back. It was no longer going to be the three of us. Work would never be the same, home life would change and the prospect of my whole life and future taking a different path in just a matter of days was really daunting.

Work was a great distraction and I worked harder than ever to try to clear down my projects, hand over to my colleagues and try to cause as little disruption to the business as possible during my week off.

I was nervous revisiting the clinic on Wednesday and had no idea what to expect from the next scan. I was still struggling with the pain and discomfort in my tummy and was still battling in my mind with wanting to progress but knowing in reality that the cost could be my health or even my life, and that of course wasn't worth the risk. By now I was feeling really poorly. As well as having extreme nausea and a severely extended stomach that ached constantly, my sore throat had also really kicked in and developed into a streaming cold. I was terrified Denise would take one look at me and deny me the transfer but I was perhaps more terrified that I could convince her otherwise by putting on a brave face when in fact I should have been honest and stopped the treatment.

As it was, the scan showed that the levels had come down and the coasting had worked, so it was go go go for Friday. We could proceed.

I have never punched the air, in my life. I thought it was something only Tom Cruise did in movies but as I walked out of the main entrance I found myself doing just that! I actually drew my arm back and with terrific force, thrust it in the air! What must I have looked like? "YES!" I could literally have burst. The potential that after all the build up, the cautiousness about the treatment itself, the drugs, the cost and then the over stimulation, we could then have been prevented from actually proceeding with the treatment, had been a huge shock to us. Feeling so poorly and so low it was extremely hard to be positive, especially with the knowledge that there was little I could do to change the situation. To know now for certain that we were going to go ahead felt utterly exhilarating. I was ecstatic!

Thursday was really, really busy at work as I was trying to hand over my projects to the team and wrap up outstanding actions. Saying good night to the team felt strange. It wasn't as if they knew what I was doing or where I was going as they had all believed I was just taking time out to spend with the family. Dom gave me a squeeze but said little and that was really helpful and sweet in a way.

It was raining so I said I'd give Emma a lift home and on the way we saw a good friend of ours so I stopped to pick him up too. He looked smart in his suit and raincoat though was starting to get drenched in the heavy rain. As I pulled up he ran to the back door of my jeep which was nearest to him and hurriedly tried to scramble into the back seat as another car pulled up right behind us. The rain was pelting down so hard and he was rushing so much to avoid delaying the growing traffic jam behind us, that he couldn't hear me shouting "other side!" as I tried to tell him Zac's car seat was blocking his way.

Instead of stopping, getting out and running round the other side, the chaos caused him to keep pushing himself and his briefcase forwards into the back seat, over Zac's car seat. To this day, that sight still makes me crack up laughing and that night in the car I nearly wet myself in hysterics! He is one of the most prominent professionals in the region, and there he was, wet through, trying to stuff himself and a briefcase into the back seat of my car, through the tiny space left above a child's car seat! All three of us howled and cried with laughter all the way to their houses as we kept reliving the story over and over again.

We dropped our friend off so now there was just Emma and I left in the car, but I continued to laugh uncontrollably. It was a strange release of a pent up tension that had been building all day and I literally could not stop laughing. After several minutes and having wiped countless tears from my eyes I then realised that I was now actually weeping, crying, sobbing in fact.

"This is it Emma". We fell silent. This really was a strange moment. I will never forget saying those exact words. From that exact moment life would never be the same again. As I left her at her house, my focus would immediately be on my family and what lay ahead tomorrow. Whilst we had been preparing for weeks, it felt that the time had now come for a gearshift and I was filled with terror at it not working and filled with anxiety about what lay ahead if it did. Either way, life was about to change and the weight of that feeling was immense.

Laughing so much had been a trigger, a very funny trigger and it was nice to laugh in a strange sort of way, but now I was terrified about turning the car round. Part of me wanted to get going but part of me was so frightened that the great white knight I had been so keen to carry me away, wasn't going to be all that he cracked up to be after all. It felt like sometimes it's best to simply retain the hope instead of rolling the dice and confirming inevitable disappointment. Keep it in the locker and you always have that hope. But now, just 12 hours to go till our appointment, there was no turning back, no denying that knight into our lives and we were about to embark on what I desperately hoped would be a thrilling adventure.

I wiped my tears, hugged Emma and drove home in silence. No phone, no radio, just me and my thoughts.

Little did I know, there was to be more hilarity later that night. After dinner Jason was a real sweetheart and offered to run me a nice bath to relax in and prepare myself for the following morning. Whilst I was downstairs in goal in front of the radiator with Zac kicking ball after ball at me, Jason went upstairs to prepare the bath. Zac was insisting that he come in the bath with Mummy and I was trying to persuade him otherwise whilst trying to catch each ball flying towards me, when Jason called me to come upstairs. The promise that Daddy would come down and go in goal, had distracted Zac from wanting to get in the bath so I was looking forward to having some peace and quiet all on my own.

Candles were lit, the bubbles were piled to the top and my fluffy dressing gown was placed across the table waiting for me. The candlelight against the travertine walls gave a lovely warm glow to the bathroom as Jason proudly walked me in. As I undressed he disappeared but quickly came back with a tall glass filled with ice and lemon. "It's a tonic darls, you'll have to pretend there's a gin in there but I've squeezed the lemon well so it should still taste lovely!"

He was so thoughtful sometimes and I felt very lucky to have such a supportive, caring husband who knew that the night before what was going be a stressful day, I needed a lovely bit of TLC and a hot, bubbly bath. Jason left and I climbed in, leaning back as the water and bubbles enveloped what was by now a huge, round, swollen tummy. Exhaling, I closed my eyes and could just hear Jason and Zac's laughter in the distance downstairs. It would all be worth it I thought as I put my head back and slowly started to relax.

And then I noticed. The bubbles were glistening. They looked really pretty, more pretty than usual and seemed to have a slight sparkle. I stroked the top of a pile of bubbles and yes; they were indeed really sparkly tonight. Oh no. I pushed the bubbles aside and looked at the water. The water seemed fine, seemed normal, but something wasn't right. I shuffled round and sat up. Sending the water swirling round me I could see that the water was glistening too! I looked up and it was then that I realised this was no ordinary bath. My bath bomb was missing from the shelf.

"Jasoooonnn!" Jason, quickly followed by Zac, ran up the stairs. Turning the light on, it was now really clear to see the beautiful effects the bath bomb had made on my bath and which had by now, covered me from head to toe in teeny, tiny, gold and pink glitter.

I knelt up and the full effect of the bath bomb could clearly be seen. The water was a pinkie colour and had tiny flakes of glitter all through it. Glitter was all over the bubbles, up the sides of the bath and worst of all, it was all over my skin! It was bloody everywhere! It was futile to ask Jason what on earth he had been thinking or to be cross, because as he said, he had seen I had a bath bomb that hadn't been used for ages and presumed I was saving it for a special occasion. In his quest to provide the perfect evening with a gorgeous bath he had inadvertently added more stress to the situation.

I tried wiping at my arms and legs but obviously the glitter just stuck or moved. When I got out of the bath I got straight into the shower, scrubbing at my skin to try to get it all off. I dragged the towel across my body but could still see tiny flecks catching the light as I moved. Three showers later, I was now tired, even more sore and by that stage past caring whether all the glitter had gone or not. Jason had emptied the bath and was completing a similar task trying to rinse all the glitter from the sides and around the plughole, with similar limited success.

In just 12 hours I was to be in a theatre, naked from the waist down, with half a dozen medical staff at my lower end and all I could think now was that they would all think I had come dressed for the occasion. That I had arranged a Vajazzle on purpose! I couldn't even bare to contemplate how much glitter would be left down, around or even up my lady bits but I was by now resigned to the fact that there was not a cat in hells chance that I would have managed to remove every single piece! Legs akimbo, theatre lights directly on me, you could be sure I'd be sparkling away tomorrow morning!

As I explained to Jason, the reason the offending bath bomb had been on the shelf for so long was that Jo had bought it for me as a present and having noted that it was glittery, I had long thought it would be too messy to use but it made a nice display item. Of all the nights for Jason to think to use it! I could hardly believe it! Laugh was all that we could do and we had to see the funny side. I'd deal with tomorrow morning when I'd be dying of embarrassment and searching faces to see if anyone noticed then, but for now I just had to call Jo and 'thank' her for her gift. How thoughtful they had both been!

Harvest time

Friday morning was so surreal. I suppose like the moment when you are just about to jump out of a plane and you have no idea what it's really going to feel like. We had read books, spoken to friends, even seen TV programmes about IVF, but really, nothing could prepare us for the experience that morning.

A cocktail of excitement, fear and of course bursting follicles meant that my stomach was in complete knots. I could hardly walk straight and as we arrived at the clinic I tried my best to stand upright in case I alerted Denise and she had second thoughts. Occasionally the thought of my decorated lady bits crept into my head, though I was more hopeful that after two further showers this morning and plenty of further douching, I may have removed any flecks that might distract the team and they wouldn't notice! It was nice to have an amusing distraction in some ways though I obviously couldn't share my concerns with the team!

Nerves made me giddy and coupled with the obvious excitement, I found myself turning into 'chatty' Helen with all the nurses, when really I should have probably kept myself to myself. The clinic's treatment area is as it should be, white, sterile and divided up with curtains. Apart from random Take That music on in the background, it is also very quiet. Unfortunately for Jason, and probably any other girl having treatment that day, this didn't stop me from being the town clown, chatting, joking away with the nurses and singing along with Gary Barlow. I couldn't help myself. I put it down to nerves.

I was given a gown and hair net and Jason too was given a hair net and shoe covers. As I ungainly climbed onto the bed, trying to minimise the immense pain in my stomach as much as possible, I could see Jason eying up his hair net. I knew what was coming next! "Do you think I really have to wear that?".

When Caroline the nurse came through moments later we both attacked poor Jason at daring to moan about wearing a hair net! That was the least he could do! It was a lovely injection of humour and distraction for us both as we laughed away and Caroline and I continued to wind Jason up.

Jason was then asked to perform, do his bit, and deliver the magic or however you want to term his input. He went off to find the room with the nurse and seemed to be away for ages! First I found it funny, then I got a bit angry at the thought of him enjoying himself or so I thought, and then I started to worry a little that he might be having a bit of trouble. As soon as his head reappeared round the curtain I was so pleased to see him back with me and delighted to hear he had 'done well'! He started squirming at the embarrassment of being led into the room and then being asked "any spillage?" Once again, his comments about his mild discomfort got little sympathy from me and he was again told that putting up with a bit of embarrassment was nothing to what I had endured. My poor husband, like he really needed that lecture at that moment but there are times and places when you really shouldn't provoke a heavily hormonal woman in pain and that was one of them!

With the canula in the back of my hand now, we were eventually shown into the small theatre adjacent to the waiting area. Again, in my naivety I was surprised that it was actually a small theatre and this terrified me! There was bed in the centre, stirrup rests and various lamps, screens and trays of steel equipment to the side. The trouble was I hadn't really imagined this scenario so whatever you had placed before me would have surprised me. I sat on the bed with Denise, various nurses, the embryologists and Jason all in the room. I signed various documents and was given a sedative and asked to lie still.

I have vague recollection of the egg retrieval and of the nurses and Jason soothing me. Though sedated it was uncomfortable and at times I would get a piercing pain in an area I couldn't really identify other than it was deep within me.

By the end of the 20 minutes they had retrieved 15 eggs, which was a very good result. The scan had shown that there were many follicles still left, the ovaries were enlarged and there was still some fluid around the ovaries which indicated the over-stimulation from before, but they had successfully retrieved sufficient quality eggs and that was now another hurdle completed.

I was returned to my private cubicle in the waiting area on the trolley as I was still pretty sedated. I lay there for some time apparently asking Jason the same questions over and over about how many eggs, how big etc? As I began to come round the pain was excruciating. Having had stomach ulcers in the past I was unable to take the recommended Ibuprofen so had just had paracetamol, but with the additional complication of the enlarged ovaries, it was just not touching the pain at all. Caroline complimented Jason on how well his hair had held up under the net and told me to get dressed but to take my time. We had a cup of tea and chocolate biscuits. Never did tea and digestives taste so good!

Yet the pain didn't appear to be subsiding. I managed to drag myself to the toilet where I threw up and then had to call Jason as I felt I might pass out. He took me back to the bed where I lay back down and went in and out of sleep or sedation. Caroline came back to check on me and though it could take some time to come round fully, she was a little surprised at how out of it I was and how much pain I was in.

Time was passing and I still felt horrendous. The pain deep inside wasn't getting any better and I felt so drunk it was starting to be a little embarrassing. By this time, we had struck up such a rapport with Caroline that we were all laughing and joking about the state I was in, but, just like when you are drunk and friends are laughing around you, it was as frustrating as it was funny.

Jason urged me to get dressed and get myself home where he felt I'd recover more quickly. The only parts of the next few hours I can remember are being almost dragged down the corridor by Jason and then unceremoniously dumped in a heap on a chair by the front door whilst he ran to get the car! Glamorous it was not!

I could do little else but rest over the weekend as I was still in a huge amount of pain and felt exhausted. We received a call to say that 14 of the eggs had fertilised so we felt delighted to be progressing and it was exciting to think about all that was happening in the lab as we carried on with our normal family life back home.

Well, as normal as family life can be with a little boy whose parents are going through IVF treatment. Time and again we had to warn Zac about going near my tummy, or I'd yell out in pain when he'd accidentally stick a sharp elbow or shoulder in me. Trying to explain to him that I wasn't ill, or in danger or that it wasn't anything for him to worry about, was tricky, as we couldn't really tell him the real reason. Most of the time, 'Mummy's got a sore tummy today' would suffice but on his more inquisitive days, playing trying to guess why Mummy's tummy is sore, was always a winner with the most outlandish answers generating hysterics from our little boy.

In brighter, less painful moments, my excitement literally wanted to boil over and tell everyone, in particular Zac, everything that we were doing. I couldn't wait to tell him but knew that there wasn't really anything to tell a four year old just yet. To think he may have a little brother or sister growing in the lab as we sat watching yet another episode of Fireman Sam, was almost too much to bear and I'd shudder with excitement. In more sombre hours, I would hold him close and slowly inhale his comforting little boy smell and pray to God he wouldn't be on his own for much longer yet giving thanks for having this funny little man in our lives already.

Some days it all got too much. I swore this would be the one and only time I could do this and that it had better bloody work because I was never going through this again. I've heard many girls say that about childbirth but Mother Nature does her crafty wand waving and makes you forget the bad bits so you want to go again. At the time I wasn't sure Mother Nature's wand was big or magic enough to make me forget this IVF cycle. Every pill, every injection, every pessary, the internal scans with what I've since heard called the 'dildo cam', the prodding, poking and all round intrusion of your most personal space and places....never mind the mental and emotional torment. I was never ever doing this again!

Five days after the egg retrieval, we woke with anticipation waiting for the call from the lab telling us whether any of our embryos had made it to the blastocyst stage. Two days earlier they had called to say that eleven were of a good enough quality to hold off transfer and wait until they had reached the next stage, which they termed blastocyst. These are more mature, more developed and stronger embryos which have a better chance of surviving and implanting, though there is a danger that they may not survive at all over the extra two days. Mine were felt to be of sufficient quality to wait for a day five transfer.

Two days later, receiving that call from the embryologist at 8.30am was yet another moment when someone's words might cause you to literally collapse with emotion. To hear that they had survived, my little embryos had made it and were ready waiting for me was almost overwhelming. "Well done little embies! I'm coming for you!" I couldn't wait to get back to them, as if they would know I was going to be there. "Thank you so so much and please look after them till I get there" I could hear myself saying to the embryologist. And then I did collapse, crying, as Jason cradled me on the landing at the top of the stairs.

Transfer day

I quickly showered and dressed as did Jason, and we could hardly speak to each other such was our excitement, nerves and anticipation. I was amused that I had dressed in fairly smart clothes but realised that indeed this was a special occasion. The way I saw it was this was the day I would first meet and get to know my new baby. What day is more special than that?

Jason took Zac to nursery whilst I carried on faffing around getting ready. I could hardly look at Zac's little face to say goodbye as it made me too nervous, too paranoid to think that I could be about to have another gorgeous baby like him. Could I really be that lucky? I cupped his cheeks in my hands and drew his face to mine whispering how much I loved him and wished him a lovely day. I could feel my throat tighten and eyes start to glisten so hurriedly gave him a squeeze and off they went out of the front door. I couldn't let him see me crying, it wasn't fair to him and there was no way I could begin to explain to my baby boy what I was feeling right at that moment.

My love for him was so great sometimes it scared me. I used to sometimes think it was perhaps the magnitude of my love for that child that ignited the longing for another. It frustrated me that I wasn't sure he knew the extent of my love for him, but he was three, he knew enough to love me back and other than that he had his toys, football and Fireman Sam to think about! To those who would repeatedly tell me I was lucky to have him, I knew that more than anyone! I bloody knew it so badly it hurt!

We were greeted at the clinic with bright smiles from the team as ever and shown to the waiting area where I undressed and prepared for theatre. We didn't have to wait long and I sat up on the bed as the team came and got me ready. Denise began to explain that whilst we had four really good blastocysts, they recommended only transferring one to be safe for baby and safe for me. Blastocysts had a tendency to split and multiple pregnancies had many risks. I had read about single embryo transfers and the increasing push to encourage them to minimise multiple pregnancies but I had a single, strong opinion on the matter from the start.

I understood the reasoning, the risk and after all, having one more baby would have fulfilled all my dreams, but if transferring two embryos increased my chances of having that one baby, then the risk of more than one baby was no risk at all. It was a bonus, would be a blessing and I was adamant that if I was lucky enough to have the choice, then I wanted to transfer two. I had known friends who had had two transferred and of those who had been successful, just as many had delivered one baby as had delivered twins. Sat there on that bed, at that moment, I wanted my very best chance and I wanted two embryos.

Denise thought differently. For the second time, her no fuss, straightforward and matter of fact approach floored me. She was adamant that their best advice was that my uterus wall lining was good; my embryo was high quality and putting one back would be most highly recommended. She added that there are many complications in a multiple pregnancy that could potentially put either or both babies at risk.

I was flung into turmoil. This was not a discussion I had expected at this time and I wasn't comfortable having it whilst sat on the bed, wearing my gown in the theatre just before the procedure. I felt hijacked. Denise, the nurses and the embryologists were all looking at us for our response but their look felt more of a telling look and I felt under immense pressure to have the single transfer. Yet it wasn't what I wanted, wasn't what I had planned to have and the uncertainty was making me panic, hyperventilate, sweat and of course cry. My head was all over the place and whilst the team were lovely and comforting I just wanted to push them away and shout, "Just put them all back and give me the best chance to have my baby!" Of course I didn't do that, I just sobbed quietly into Jason's shoulder and hid my face at the shame I felt in what seemed like my naivety at the situation. I just wanted a baby. I wasn't greedy, I wasn't trying to be the next Octomum and I was definitely not trying to defy the far greater knowledge and expertise of this amazing team, but I knew I was also not really happy in just having one embryo transferred.

And so, we had one embryo transferred. Of course we did! I took their best advice and once we confirmed we would just transfer one, I immediately felt a little calmer and more confident as we got back on track and got on with the procedure. I just wanted a baby.

The embryologist put the embryo onto a screen in the corner of the room and the sight of those cells took my breath away. "Hello baby" I whispered and squeezed Jason's hand as we both stared at the new life being created. It was amazing. I was surprised at how I immediately felt a yearning to be closer to it, to care for it and to be responsible for it. I was hugely excited as they checked all the data to confirm it was definitely our embryo and then brought the pipette through from the lab to the theatre.

Nothing ever runs smoothly for me and despite having had a smooth rehearsal of the transfer some weeks earlier, it appeared that I had a kink in my cervix which Denise described as a corkscrew shape and so the catheter they use to insert the embryos had trouble reaching the top of the cervix and into the uterus. After several attempts, Denise changed the catheter to a softer tube and eventually, our little 'emby' was transferred back to Mummy.

In recovery where I was told to rest for an hour, I held my palms across my tummy with utter contentment. I was talking to it in my head, soothing it, loving it and anyone watching me not knowing the circumstances would surely have thought I'd gone mad. Jason too was calmer now and we both sat, holding hands, touching my tummy and dreaming of what was to come.

The embryologist came to see us and explained that we had three excellent blastocysts remaining and asked us if we had thought about freezing any. We hadn't dared to dream that any would make it to transfer, let alone freeze additional ones so she talked us through it all, read all the formalities and we discussed the options. Overwhelmingly, given my sensitivity to the drugs and hyper stimulation, it was felt that should this round not work, I could avoid that stimulation stage next time and therefore be healthier for the transfer. This made sense but it was the optimism that we could have another child, or perhaps two, after this one that made me really decide to freeze them. I could hardly contemplate for a second that this treatment would fail. Such negative, defeatist thoughts were banned from forming in or entering my head, but yes, we agreed to freeze them to keep our options open for the future.

The two-week wait

Any self-help book, blog or website describes how utterly horrid the two week wait from transfer to pregnancy test is and yet none can ever really, fully describe how really horrendous it is for a couple. Your mind plays tricks, your body plays tricks and your thoughts are 100% consumed by the prospect of being pregnant or the possibility that you are not. It's like walking round with a brick wall in front of your face that you can't see through, round, or over. It's ever present from the moment you rouse in the morning with your head still on the pillow; to the moment you finally find sleep at night.

Every twinge in your tummy, tweak of your boobs, taste, smell, ache sends your mind into overdrive. "Am I?", "Could I be", "I've never felt like this before", "I just can't be"... and so it goes on. One minute you are cast iron convinced you are definitely pregnant and start working out due dates on Pampers' online calculator and the next you are in deep despair convinced you're not and trying to decide whether to have a commiserating glass of wine to make you feel better, until that flurry of hope that you still could be, kicks in and stops you.

Should I?, Shouldn't I?, Am I?, Aren't I?, I am, I am? I'm totally not!.....

And if it's not hard enough reading into everything yourself, you have close family and friends reading into everything you do. Telling you your boobs have never looked that big, your skin looks glowing, or that because they remember you once eating and enjoying a tuna melt and now you don't fancy it, you must be pregnant!

The two-week wait is often described as agony because that's exactly what it is. There is simply nothing you can do but wait, but if only you could just wait and not analyse or think. If you could switch off your senses and imagination that would be perfect and the wait would be easy. But nobody said having a baby was easy and definitely nobody said having a baby through IVF was going to be easy.

I was instructed to insert three large white vaginal pessaries each evening before I went to bed. Injections were horrid, internal scans were invasive but nothing beats the vaginal pessary for being the most degrading aspect of the whole process. I used to sneer at them, calling them the Devil's eggs, almost as if they could hear me and I could vent a little frustration at each one! I hated them with such a passion. Each night, I'd hide away in the ensuite and try to ram all three up so that I could be comfortable in bed and each night I'd curse under my breath at the indignity of doing so. How unladylike. Holy cow, surely someone could invent another means of getting this bloody drug inside you? For some reason, doing this each night made me furious and worse still was the following day, when the remnants of the pessary would often refuse to flush away down the toilet. Every time you go to pee, a thick creamy white paste would float on the surface of the toilet and it took great effort and tricks with toilet paper to ensure you got it all away. At work, this was a constant stress and one again that would infuriate me. Zac had noticed a few times and would shout out "What's this toothpaste doing in the toilet Mummy?" I tutted, blamed Daddy and quickly tried to distract my very observant little boy! Each time I thought about the flipping pessaries the same words would always enter my head "As if you don't go through enough!" It was disgusting!

By now, my cold had also developed into a full blown chest infection so I felt dreadful as I tried to relax and forget about the wait and impending results. I coughed my way through each day and my body felt heavy as I desperately tried hard to be positive and chirpy on my return to work.

It's hard enough to drag yourself through each day at work when you feel so poorly, but the emotional drain from the previous week had obviously sapped my body of any energy reserves and I felt shocking.

As is my usual way, I threw myself into work, giving my all, trying to pull myself through the illness and forget about the wait. Work had always been my saviour and we were really busy so my clients were my distraction, which made me feel much better. I still felt excited and my tummy was turning at the anticipation, but throwing myself into client meetings and working with our team in the office would be all the distraction I needed to help the clock whizz by.

On the Monday, the first day back in the office, I had a meeting in the afternoon just round the corner from the office at one of my favourite clients. I'd worked with the guys for years and felt really comfortable with them and loved the work we were doing for them. I was to go on my own for this meeting and so I left our team's weekly huddle meeting early, to pop to the loo for a quick wee before I headed out the door.

Blood. I was bleeding. I checked again and there it was, blood mixed with clear mucus. But it was definitely blood. What the hell did that mean? My head was spinning, I felt faint and suddenly felt really, really hot. I felt like I wanted to cry, but I wasn't really sure why or what I would be crying for. I struggled to get my head straight, aware that I needed to get to my meeting but half thinking I would have to cancel as I didn't know how I was going to get out of the toilet never mind to their offices. I couldn't call out to anyone in the office, phone anyone, or do anything at all other than check again. Once again, I stared at the blood stained paper in disbelief.

No! No, no, no, this couldn't be happening. But it was happening and I had a meeting in 5 minutes. I had no idea how the hell I could explain to my team or my client why all of a sudden I couldn't make it, so would have to go. Shit!

I sorted myself out and headed out the door shouting "bye" to the team and avoiding putting my head into the meeting room to say I was going. I walked as fast as I could to the meeting, trying to avoid having any time on my own that would allow my mind to wander and think about what had just happened. I just wanted to get to the meeting, start talking and get it over with as quickly as possible.

Sometimes you are able to do amazing things in the most extraordinary of circumstances and getting through that meeting, whilst giving a sterling performance I might add, was one of them!

I literally ran out of the client's office, bolted down the stairs instead of using the lift and slumped against the wall of the alley immediately next to their building. I rang the clinic. I can't remember the details of the conversation but in essence it went something like this:

"I'm bleeding"

"I'm sorry"

There was of course much more to it than that and a lot more said between us, but it was the nurse's succinct words of "I'm sorry" as a response that always stuck in my head. So I'm not pregnant then? It is all over? That's it, no hope, no maybes, and no potentially positive explanation? I've lost it and I'm not having a baby?

They told me to see how I went throughout the day and call back tomorrow if the bleed continued.

Shock does strange things to the body and at that moment I thought I might faint, have a heart attack, poo myself, or all three at once. I had visions of who might find me in the alleyway and wondered how on earth I might explain my predicament if all three did in fact happen. I was instantly terrified of what might immediately become of me as I stood there, stooping, holding the wall gasping for breath and trying to compose myself. I just wanted to be at home, I wanted Jason, I wanted my Mum. I needed someone to scoop me up and hold me, whilst I let my body crumble and the tear floodgates open. What the hell was I going to do now? I started to worry whether my legs would hold me up?

I couldn't go to my car and drive home as my keys were on my desk so I slowly made my way back to the office. Every slow step seemed to take forever and I realised that even though that was the only place I could possibly go, I really wasn't ready to face anyone.

Halfway back I stumbled onto a low wall beside a car park and broke down crying. Oh God I wasn't pregnant, how could this be true? I phoned Jo and as soon as I said "Hi" my voice cracked and I cried down the phone telling her that I was bleeding. In a way I felt immediate sympathy for Jo because I knew that she too would be broken hearted and the poor girl had to try to console me, when there was no real consolation. She let me cry, showed me sympathy and also picked me up by telling me that bleeds were common in the early stages. I had unfortunately left my notes from the clinic at home and so wasn't able to read up on their advice about aftercare or signs to look out for. Talking to Jo about it and having a really good cry helped get the sorrow, panic and anxiety out of my system a little, which in turn helped me to pull myself together a bit better. Jo suggested I read through my notes that evening and see if they mentioned anything about early bleeds and try to rest for the remainder of the day. Turning off my phone I had another brief cry, blew my nose, took a deep breath and headed back to the office. Brave face on, normality needed to resume.

I couldn't phone Jason yet. I hadn't got my own head round it yet and wasn't in a fit state to try to tell him whilst being coherent. It would just end up being a wail and he certainly didn't need that when he was no doubt driving on the motorway somewhere between dealerships as he often was. I needed to make sense of it first and try to get my own head round it so I could tell him in a way that he could then deal with and digest the information, rather than have him leap into panic mode too. It might sound strange that I wouldn't tell him immediately but there have been very few times in my life when I have let rip with anxiety at those closest to me, either down the phone or in person. I have always been a fixer, the one that copes and always hated passing on any worry. Telling Jo was different as she was one step, even though a tiny step, away from the situation, but it would really have taken something hugely traumatic and left me helpless, for me to knee-jerk react and phone my Mum or Jason on anything that I thought would be upsetting.

When I finally made my way back into the office, clearly one look at my face showed that all was not well. As I stood warming myself against the radiator opposite Emma's desk I was thankful for it's stability as well as it's warmth as I held onto it and then broke down telling her I was bleeding. I'm sure there was a part of her that was immediately thankful I wasn't crying due to something going dramatically wrong in the meeting, as would have been my initial reaction, but she took me in her arms and I literally shook with shock and grief.

I simply couldn't believe the words I was saying. Surely not? Not more than an hour before I was well on my way to having a baby. I was bouncing round the office, whilst the team were unaware I was cooking a baby and I felt really excited. Now, barely lunchtime and it was all over. End of everything.

That afternoon, myself, Emma and Dom were due to have an off site management strategy meeting discussing the direction and focus for the business for the next 12 months. It had been a long-standing date in the diary and as it was often difficult to get us all together for any length of time for these meetings we were reluctant to reschedule. At that moment, however I was of no use to anyone, let alone to be thinking strategically and making important business and financial decisions. There is never a good time, but this was really not a good time. I just wanted to run, to drive away, to go home, curl up and cry.

And yet, as ever, work needed to be my saviour. I decided to call the clinic again first and get some clarity on what they thought as I could remember nothing from my initial conversation. This time, a little better prepared I explained the type of bleed and spoke to a different nurse. It was true, it wasn't a great sign, but within this timeframe it was quite common to have a 'show' or bleed which could signify implantation. If the implantation of the embryo into the uterus wall lining was particularly aggressive this could cause a small bleed and this could be a good sign, especially if the 'show' was mucusy, which it had been. The advice was to relax, rest a little and wait and see what happened over the next few days.

I didn't feel I'd bounced back and I didn't feel positive but I felt there was a little hope and with that, I was a little more buoyed than I had been earlier. I walked back into the office feeling more like myself and feeling that an off site planning meeting was perfectly timed, especially as we were to have lunch too!

The meeting was exactly what I needed to stop the tears, stop the worry and try to relax a little about it all. I told Dom as we walked across to the hotel where we were to meet and after that nothing was mentioned between the three of us. Occasionally I would get a twinge or a stabbing pain as sitting on the low Chesterfield sofa wasn't great for my bloated, tender tummy but apart from that we had a great meeting and came away with loads of decisions made.

I collected Zac from nursery and as soon as I saw him I could feel my eyes starting to burn. He was chatting away about his friends Harry, Eva and Lydia, and even though I was listening, I had a strange, distracted feeling that I was holding back from blurting out an apology to him. It was so surreal. Here I was, with my beloved child, who was fit, healthy and hilarious and who was gushing to tell me all about his lovely day and yet I wasn't enjoying his moment. I didn't know whether I wanted to apologise for feeling so down and distracted by the events of my day, or to apologise for potentially not being pregnant.

I looked down at his gorgeous, happy little face as we got to the car and knew I just had to shake off the negativity somehow or many more special moments like this with him would pass and I wouldn't even notice. As ever, scooping him up and giving him a squeeze did wonders for my mood. Between us we had developed the most gorgeous cuddle that we called 'cheek to cheek' that, even without little arms around my neck, was the most unbelievable tonic for any mood. When he stopped tearing round the house like a tornado and came to place his soft little cheek against mine, it brought an instant calm and made my heart burst. It was always a feeling I never wanted to end and seemed to make everything all right with the world.

That evening as we walked in the door I went straight to my notes from the clinic. There was a short paragraph about potential spotting being normal and I felt a little more reassured.

Telling Jason was hard, as I knew the pain and shock he was feeling but it also brought out a little positivity in me as I drew strength in trying to reassure him it could be normal and a good sign. I wasn't sure what to believe but I knew I wished I wasn't bleeding. Aside from the drugs, you also need hope when undergoing IVF and at that moment, hope was all I felt I had left.

Testing, testing...

Throughout the two-week wait you are desperate to do a pregnancy test but you are always advised not to do so until day 14. Day 14 was Thursday and Emma and I were due at an all day client strategy meeting across on the Wirral, literally the other side of the country. If I were to do the test that morning, whatever the outcome, I would be in no fit state to lead the meeting that was planned with the three Board Directors of a brand new client.

By Tuesday I was still bleeding. By Wednesday, I could wait no longer. It was Day 12. Waking that morning, I was still showing blood but the flow had slowed and I was in a little less pain. Jason and I discussed long and hard about whether or not to do the test a day early and in the end decided that Thursday was not an option and waiting until Friday was probably not worth the additional anxiety. I was still bleeding which didn't seem positive. So, we decided that we would do the test that morning.

I had already spoken to Emma and Dom the night before and said I wouldn't be in the office that following day and would work from home as much as I could. I was on my knees still with the horrendous chest infection, hardly sleeping, my chest was aching and my headache hadn't shifted for days. Thursday's meeting was really important to the agency and I needed to try to get stronger for that, and whatever the result of the test, I couldn't see myself coping in front of the team in the office, especially feeling so weak and run down.

That morning, it was the strangest mix of emotions I think I had and will ever feel. Jason and I had sat in our bathroom many times and literally done dozens of pregnancy tests in there over the years and each time we had sat there feeling optimistic, almost giddy but always tinged with a last little bit of doubt that we constantly retained out of self preservation. If we ever actually got to the stage of doing a test, it had always meant that we had gone through days of waiting for a period that never came and possibly some other symptoms so it always meant that we were convinced we had a good chance of a positive result.

This time was different. I had been bleeding for two days since Monday and that couldn't be a good sign. We needed to do the test to confirm that I wasn't but we both still had a twinge of optimism that perhaps we could still be pregnant after all, and the bleed was just an aggressive implantation. It was almost as if the balance of emotions involved had been completely reversed this time as I tentatively peed on the stick and we waited for the result. As usual we had bought one of the fail safe, expensive smiley face digital tests rather than the cheap and cheerful double line sticks. When we found out we were pregnant with Zac, I peed on four sticks to check we could actually make out the double lines before Jason dashed out to Boots to get a digital smiley version just to check for certain. I remember the doctor making me feel silly when she said: "I won't bother testing you, I'm sure after 5 tests we can pretty much say for certain that you're pregnant don't you? Don't bother buying any more."

I always struggled to leave the ensuite and not peak at the test. I tried going back into the bedroom like Jason but felt I needed to be there as soon as the time was up. When time was eventually up, Jason wasn't in the bathroom, so I still couldn't look. After nagging him to quickly come back we stood there holding hands. I was holding the stick and we stared into each other's faces. I was desperate to look but too nervous to at the same time.

It was positive.

It was bloody positive! What? It really was smiling back at me. One quick check of the box to double check this was what the result meant and yes, it was. It was bloody smiling back at us! We were pregnant!

We couldn't believe it. Literally couldn't believe what we were seeing. Of course I did a second and the second confirmed the same result. After all the worry and anxiety of the last couple of days we were so relieved to have ended all that heartache and done the test a day early. I was ecstatic, over the moon and yet part of me was still trying to switch my brain into positive giddy mode. It was an amazing feeling. I just wanted to scream from the top of my lungs, but of course, I couldn't. We had a little boy to get up and ready for nursery and needed to remain as normal as possible for his sake.

I was desperate to run into his room. Desperate to squeeze him and tell him, to share our family's great news. As it was he dragged his tired little, half awake body into our doorway just at that moment and my 'sensible mum' head kicked in as I scooped him up, hugged him and took him downstairs for his breakfast before he got too grumpy!

When Jason left for work taking Zac with him to drop off at nursery, I called the clinic and advised them of our result. I felt immense shame at admitting to have done the test a day early and was aware that my nerves were making me ramble on with excuses about why I had ignored all advice and not waited another day. As I was still bleeding they asked me to go to the clinic for a blood test to check my HCG levels, which I did later that afternoon.

I was still feeling truly shocking, really poorly given the positive result, yet I was excited as I dragged myself to the hospital for the blood test. I think I was expecting more from the visit but as it was I just sat on a chair, arm on a pillow, had my blood taken and then it was time to go. They would call me the next day with the results. It felt like somewhat of an anti-climax after the excitement of the morning. I think I was perhaps expecting people to talk to me about my pregnancy, my impending baby but as it was, it was quick in and out and not even an immediate positive result to get me giddy!

The next day, Thursday I woke early, still feeling horrendously poorly, and I did another pregnancy test. After all, this was Day 14 and the day I should have actually tested in the first place. This test was one that actually said the word 'pregnant' and yup, there it was, the lovely word 'pregnant' staring back at us, once again confirming a positive result. As I dressed in the dark for our early start out to our Wirral meeting, I felt really giddy, which when combined with the ongoing bleeding and a raging cold, made for a peculiar mix of emotions so early in the morning.

Denise was due to call today with the results from yesterday's blood test. I was on tenterhooks all morning across the long drive and was really hoping that she would call before the meeting started but on the other hand was desperate to get to the meeting and get it started before she did call so I could concentrate on the job in hand, just in case the news wasn't positive. I must have chewed Emma's ear off for the entire length of the M62 that morning about the 'what, ifs, buts and maybes' of all the connotations that that day's news could possibly bring.

As it was, Denise called just as we approached the client's office and fortunately confirmed that the HCG levels were high which was a good sign.

Throughout the IVF process one aspect you quickly get used to is that with every positive result and hurdle overcome there is also a 'however' or 'but' to quickly follow as there are many more hurdles ahead of you. My initial blood test showed a positive result however, I would need a further test 48 hours later to see if the levels were climbing as they should, which would indicate a pregnancy. So, despite reading high now which was a good sign, this first reading should really be seen as just a yardstick. But, as I had become adept at doing, I pulled it back to the here and now and focussed on the fact that it was definitely another hurdle overcome and the positive result that we wanted.

Friday came and I had gone rapidly downhill with my chest infection. I had been up all night coughing and by morning, could hardly lift my head from the pillow. Thursday had been a long, gruelling day and really I probably should have cancelled that meeting that I'd coughed all the way through. Plus we were too polite to admit we'd not had lunch and so from an early start we'd eaten nothing until after 6pm when we pulled into a McDonalds and rammed 20 chicken nuggets down us! Tasty but hardly looking after ourselves! I was really paying the price now. I had an appointment at the clinic for a follow up blood test first thing. I popped into the office for my files and took them home to work on the sofa, where I could cough and bark to my heart's content without bothering anyone else.

Denise had promised to try to get the bloods rushed through and get the results back to us later that day, but if not it could be Saturday or potentially Monday. Jason was planning on trying to get back early and finish his work in his office at home to be here when they called, so another reason I hoped it would be later that day. By this time, after a turbulent week when my body felt like it was at war with itself, I didn't have a clue what the results would be. My body felt alien to me anyway given how poorly I was and with the emotional drain, I struggled to draw any strength to think cohesively or draw any conclusions as to whether I was pregnant or not.

Denise's call came earlier than expected, just after lunch. My levels had increased with the positive test; she could confirm we were pregnant. We were definitely pregnant!

I can only describe my feelings at that moment as like that of a deflating beach ball. I was deliriously ecstatic but that piece of good news was like a pin to a ball that over the last two weeks had built up with hope, anxiety, worry, excitement and positive thinking, that now could be released with the knowledge and joy that the unknown was all over. We were pregnant! I was exhausted with it all and with that final bit of news could now let it all go. I'm sure if I had the strength I would be dancing round the room but as it was, I just sat on the sofa, with my laptop warming my knees and an abundance of used snotty tissues scattered round me and cried my eyes out.

I immediately rang Jason, who whooped down the phone and said he was racing to get back home as quickly as possible. I rang my mum and cried the words down the phone to her. I could hardly believe what I was saying!

Slowly, very slowly, it started to sink in and I started to let myself believe the words; I'm pregnant. My tummy started to flutter and I remember I kept gasping to myself each time the thought came over me.

I was beyond giddy just half an hour later. I was so overjoyed and wanted to scream and tell the world. Sadly however, my body had other ideas as my headache was pounding, my hacking chest was burning and now I had developed a terrific earache, which I'd never experienced in my life before.

The day before I had taken a photograph of the pregnancy stick and now, I went into my phone photo library and stared at the photo again. 'Pregnant' it said. Eight delightful, little letters in an order that was the answer to all our prayers.

I texted Jo the photo and waited. I was smiling to myself as I did it, imagining her at the other end and how she might react. I felt like a little minx but I felt so giddy it didn't matter. Within seconds my phone was ringing and 'Jo Mobile' flashed up. She was beyond excited and said she had been walking down a corridor at work and had to leap into a meeting room to explode and then call me! Hilarious and how lovely to think of her like that!

Next I texted Emma at work and waited. Once again, as I smiled and waited, the phone rang immediately. She was walking quickly back to the office in the rain and was now walking slowly, crying into the phone after seeing the photo! What fantastic news!

Andrew, Kate, Minnie and Mum were coming up to ours for the weekend the following day, so I didn't call Andrew and waited to tell them face-to-face. There was of course still the matter of the ongoing bleeding which remained at the back of my mind as I began to think about telling more people our positive news. Jo and Emma had gone through our roller coaster week at first hand and knew we were going for all the tests that week so I felt I should and owed it to them to tell them but I was still nervous about the bleeding and what this could mean.

That evening however, I was just too excited not to tell some of our closest friends. I called them and said the same to each one when they asked how I was: "you better start knitting!" In turn, their shrieks of delight down the phone made me roar laughing and their giddiness rubbed off on me as I started to enjoy our news myself! To each one however, I heard myself saying we still had a long way to go and that I was bleeding so had to take care. Just as with every stage of IVF, with every celebration, there is also a dampener. Was I telling them or telling myself? I recall thinking it was a funny thing to say "but for now I am pregnant", but that was how it felt and yet no matter how precarious or worrying our situation was, I couldn't hold the news in any longer.

Andrew and Kate arrived really late on Friday evening so I waited until Saturday morning. The four of us were in the kitchen when I looked at Jason for reassurance that it was OK to say. "We're pregnant!" The look on both their faces was brilliant, but again, they too became subdued when I told them about the bleeding and the details of the last fortnight we'd endured.

As we all ate brunch and Zac and Minnie played together, we all kept catching each other's eyes and grinning or we'd have the occasional squeeze when we walked past one another. The excitement had lifted my mood but it hadn't lifted my chest infection and the pain in my left ear was by now excruciating. Everything in my body ached from either the infection, the IVF drugs or now I thought probably, my pregnancy.

Adjusting to life being pregnant

The family all made a trip into town that Saturday afternoon and I decided to go to the pharmacy to try to get something for my ear. By now I couldn't walk straight and could hardly hear and was almost crying with the pain. Jason took me to see the Pharmacist and we were like kids squirming with excitement as I explained my symptoms and that I was pregnant. He was lovely explaining that there was very little I could take but I wasn't really listening. I already knew that, but just loved the fact that we could tell someone officially that I was pregnant. At lunch, the pain was too much to bear so we had to leave the restaurant early and come straight home. Before I climbed into bed early that night, I checked and confirmed that I was still bleeding. And yet, I'd told my family, some friends and I'd even had an official conversation with a professional about my condition today so I put my head on the pillow, smiling as the thought that I was definitely pregnant sank in and let sleep take me.

The following morning I felt even more dreadful. We had guests and Zac had his best friend Harry's birthday party to go to, so I dragged myself downstairs to make an appearance and tried my best to get into gear, ready to enjoy the day with the family. Jason put the kettle on and I curled up on the sofa next to Mum, watching the children play in front of us. Jason took one look at me and told me to go back to bed and rest. After sleeping for another couple of hours, I got up once more but now with the most horrendous period pain. The dragging pain I'd had for more than a week was now replaced with a really sharp, intense pain deep in my abdomen. I again curled up next to Mum on the sofa with a screaming migraine and aching belly. The kids continued to play oblivious, Andrew and Kate discreetly busied themselves around the house and I could tell that Mum and Jason were trying to balance concern for me whilst making things seem as normal as possible for everyone there.

Five minutes later though, things could not have been any further from normal. With shooting pains in my stomach I decided to go to the toilet and it was there that I finally lost my pregnancy. The blood flowed thick and fast and then suddenly I passed a huge mucusy blood clot, the size of a walnut and it plopped loudly into the toilet. I cried out for Jason and Mum and could hear myself wailing, "I've lost it, I've lost it, I'm so sorry, it's gone, it's gone, I'm so sorry, I've lost it."

I pushed past them both and ran to the kitchen to get a ladle of all things, to scoop up the loss to take to the clinic. I was positive it was over, but the IVF process had drilled hope into me so deeply, that I needed to cling onto something and if taking this to show them might make them tell me there was another explanation, then that was enough for me to cling on to. And yet, deep within me, I knew. What was there was gone. What had given a positive reading was now no longer in me. Whatever stage it had gotten to, it was now over.

I felt like every ounce of my body was breaking, not just my heart.

With the pain in my belly and an intense ache in my chest I stayed on the toilet groaning with both Jason and Mum hugging me. Mum put her arm round Jason too and that gesture broke my heart further. My poor, poor husband was so upset too. It was our pregnancy but it was my body and I just wanted him to know that I was so sorry I had lost it. I was so utterly sorry that I couldn't hold onto it. A futile apology and one that he stoically told me I should not repeat, but I had such a helpless, useless feeling and I really did feel that I had let the family down.

I needed to get off the loo and get Zac ready for his party in the village hall. Of course Jason said there was no way I was going and as it turned out Andrew, Kate and Mum took him to the party and out for tea, to give Jason and I some space. I was really grateful but I didn't want to be left on my own to talk it over with Jason and I didn't want my baby boy to go to his best friend's party without his mummy. I couldn't let Zac see me in the state I was in and I certainly wasn't up to seeing anyone at a four year old's party but it didn't stop me really wanting to take him. I saw sense and let the family take him out, trying my best to talk up how exciting it was for Grandma to be taking him and for Minnie to meet his friends rather than Mummy coming. As ever, a child's resilience is amazing and he quickly forgot I wouldn't be going, which was in some ways even more hurtful! It was lose-lose for mummy however he responded!

We cried, we held each other and we put the kettle on. It was nice to have the house to ourselves but suddenly the empty house filled with grief seemed enormous with just Jason and I in it. We had a telephone number for the clinic for emergency situations where you speak to the nurse on call. We sat and wrote out all the questions we had and decided that this felt enough of an emergency to us to call the number.

For some strange reason we knelt on the floor to make the call and as Denise answered, we explained all that had happened. She confirmed our worst fear that she was pretty sure we had lost the pregnancy but that they would book us in for a scan to confirm first thing the following morning.

I had had a couple of hours to think about it and with her words of confirmation that it was all over, somehow my recovery started to kick in immediately and my attention turned to what would happen next. Amazingly I had forgotten my words of only a week ago, when I was adamant I'd never do the treatment again, and began processing when I could start a new cycle. I rattled off a dozen questions about whether I needed a D&C, how long would this period last and many more, but all I really wanted to know was when could we try again. I asked all these questions of Denise but she exercised a skill she had obviously mastered over the years when dealing with disappointed clients and focussed me on what was immediately happening on that day. We could discuss and deal with a potential second round once I had really recovered from this round. She was right but I was frustrated. I wanted to be pregnant, I wasn't pregnant right here and now so what were we going to do to ensure that I was going to be as quickly as possible. This was typical of my 'can do, will do' attitude and impatience wanting to just crack on with something, but I was underestimating the enormity of the emotional and physical recovery that I needed to go through to get me to that next positive stage.

When my family arrived back from the party and dinner, all I wanted to do was to hold Zac. I had an overwhelming desire to apologise to him as I had to Jason. I had done so much, it had all hurt so bad and yet still, I hadn't managed to give him a brother or sister. It was heart breaking to have to hold all that emotion in and ignore my own feelings as I put on a brave face to listen to his excited yet tired ramblings about the party and going to the big boy's pub where Uncle Andrew had a dirty beer! It was right that he was blissfully unaware, unfazed by his parents not going with him and oblivious to my now pale but blotchy and swollen face. Mum, Andrew and Kate all hugged us both in turn and said they were sorry. Again I felt it was I who should be sorry, but I appreciated the warmth of their hugs.

The following morning we arrived at the clinic and were greeted by a very sympathetic Denise for our scan. I gave her the sample pot which she gave a courteous glance before saying she didn't need to see anything and we would just look at the scan.

The scan showed a black blob. Apparently it was an indication of an embryonic sack so there either was a sack still there or it was a sign that there had been a sack there. It was 50:50. The loss could be explained by the transplanted embryo splitting into two, with one of the two being rejected. It was a possibility. Again our spirits were lifted. Seemingly, although very slim, there was a chance I could still be pregnant!

Denise has a great skill in only ever talking about the facts at that moment in time. There was a black blob. It was a sign of an embryonic sack. It was too early to confirm via the scan and we needed a blood test to be 100% sure. Again, with two blood tests taken 48 hours apart, we should see a rise in HCG to still have a positive pregnancy but a fall in level would indicate there was no longer a pregnancy. And so, I had further blood taken with an appointment made for Wednesday for the second test and we left the clinic.

We felt odd in a weird sort of limbo again. Yet we knew. We had both seen what I had lost the day before and we both knew that the size of it and the significant bleed meant it was almost impossible for there to be anything left. It was over. We just needed to go through the motions for confirmation. It was cruel that our recovery couldn't start until the second set of blood test results and it was even more cruel that our minds started to play tricks on us about all sorts of possibilities and explanations. By the time the second bloods were taken and the negative result confirmed, both Jason and I were so relieved that this stage was now finally over. We had lost it and our first attempt had failed. We were not pregnant now. We had to get used to that idea.

Picking ourselves up

As we started to pick ourselves up I quickly began to grow increasingly impatient. Whilst the clinic insist on only talking to you about the here and now and never want to discuss the future stages, my need to plan and know when we could go again only sought to generate massive frustration. I was to learn that the clinic needs to encourage clients to just consider the immediate stage, as there is so much to take in and deal with that if they allowed my mind to race ahead, I would only forget all the detail anyway. I guess it was some sort of preservation strategy but when Little Miss Eager Pants kicked in again and Jason and I decided we were definitely going to try again, I wanted to crack on and know the specific dates for the next round of treatment.

We had drawn strength and positivity that we had clearly been pregnant, so using this course of IVF treatment did work for us, but it was, as is so commonly said, just Mother Nature's way that this pregnancy was simply not meant to be. We took comfort in the thoughts that losing a pregnancy in this way so early was actually very common and that a number of friends and family had suffered miscarriages following natural conceptions. Sadly they were quite common and were unrelated to IVF. It was simply just not meant to be and we had to take additional comfort that it could have happened had we conceived without the treatment. It was small comfort as we had still lost our dream, but it did make us feel extremely positive about our prospects for success if we did the treatment again.

I still felt really poorly and needed to rest to try to shake off the chest and ear infections so took the remainder of the week off. Going back to work on the Monday was really hard. I tried to act normal and forget about it, but I was hyperactive, bouncing off all the walls and I was also extremely stroppy. I knew what I was like but just couldn't help it, I couldn't calm down. It was like the most extreme PMT I had ever experienced. The team had been told what had happened as apparently some had been concerned by recent comings and goings and some had actually asked Emma and Dom if I had cancer or some other horrendous condition, so I agreed that they could be told so as not to worry unnecessarily. They had however been told not to talk to me about it, which was a strange feeling but I was extremely grateful that I could get through each day without them bringing it up. For once I could keep something personal to me, which helped me focus on work until home time. Mid afternoon on that first Monday back, I was in the meeting room with Emma when I suddenly cracked. She had mentioned how I was acting and put an arm round me and I could hold back no longer. I was so sorry to be acting like that, so sorry to be creating such an atmosphere in the small confines of the office but I was even more sorry that I was helpless to change my behaviour. I was simply trying to get through the day.

We now had to tell the handful of friends that I had phoned less than a week ago to tell them the news. It was heartbreaking all over again just saying the words and I was also sad that I had made them sad, knowing how much those few people knew how badly we had wanted that baby. I quickly started saying 'don't worry, it's just shit, that's all' as I tried to stem the stream of superlatives that flow too easily from any of us when we are faced with consoling someone.

"At least you have Zac" became a much over-used and unwanted expression during those early days. Yes…. And…. So….? Yes I have Zac but I was expecting a brother or sister for him and now I'm not! I was kindly advised "not to put myself through it", to "focus on Zac" and "look after the little boy I have". I get it but I didn't understand it. I would, and felt like I had, put myself through anything for my family and that included loving Zac so much that I would go through all of this to give him a brother or sister. I was doing it because I was focussed on him and looking after him, not in spite of. It all felt so unfair that because I had been unsuccessful with my treatment, I should now consider that Zac was enough and should remain an only child. Would people have said that if I'd naturally conceived and lost my pregnancy?

One lovely friend sent a card and wrote about how brave she thought I had been to attempt the treatment. I questioned that word, as it wasn't brave as I saw it. Brave? Really? I wanted a brother or sister for Zac and this was one way of getting it, there was nothing brave in that? Yet as the days passed and I weighed up the pain of the first cycle whilst contemplating a second, I realised that actually you do need to be strong to go through IVF treatment and I started to understand and appreciate her words. You did need to be brave, you needed to dig deep to pick yourself up to have a go, despite knowing, that as well as needing all elements of the treatment to be successful, you also needed Mother Nature on your side and a truck load of luck too. Only the brave or desperate would put themselves in such a potentially painful situation.

You also need cash. We hadn't reckoned on the first time not working, on needing to write another cheque, on spending more of our savings. We had the money and for that I knew we were exceptionally fortunate but that was our security, our future for our family. Yet it was now clear that if we wanted that family we had dreamed of, we needed to write another cheque for another four-figure sum.

It seems people have very different coping techniques and at that time, anything anyone suggested to help me recover just wasn't my way. If anything, some of the suggestions infuriated me, as they seemed to show naivety or lack of understanding. In fact it was very difficult to suggest anything that would actually make me feel better and it was unfair to judge family and friends for simply trying to help.

It was November and already everyone was starting to talk about Christmas. Zac's birthday was Christmas Eve so December was always really busy for us and especially me, organising his party. All the school and nursery Christmas parties, combined with my usual last minute arrangements, meant that each year I struggled to secure entertainers for Zac's party and this year was no exception.

Lots of family and friends were all saying the same thing: "focus on Zac's birthday and Christmas, get them out of the way and see how you feel in the New Year." This only infuriated me. It was impossible to focus on Zac's birthday, I didn't care whether we had Christmas or not and I already knew now how I would bloody well feel in the New Year, and that was exactly how I felt right now! Upset. Frustrated. Desperate to get pregnant. How could I think about or enjoy anything else when I felt so broken, useless and utterly miserable? None of those events would be tonics, none of them would take the hurt away and I was pretty sure none of them would make me pregnant! They were a distraction, a mask to hide the hurt but it was ridiculous to think they could take my mind off what I felt was really important or make me feel any better at all.

Waiting any length of time seemed futile. Waiting was just another cycle lost, another month older and another month I had to look at Zac playing on his own and the gap between him and any potential sibling increasing. It wasn't an option. I knew what we wanted and I knew I had to crack on. Focussing on the second round was my only salvation and tonic. Re-focussing on anything else just made me feel more helpless and desperate.

Just as I was trying to cope, I was dealt another blow. Without going into the detail, someone close to me, that would need my support, had found herself with an unwanted pregnancy. Friends got together to tell me face to face, that she was pregnant, her boyfriend absolutely didn't want the baby and that she was going to have an abortion.

I sat back absorbing the news. Firstly the shock that she was pregnant, secondly that she was in such a horrid situation and then, obviously what she was intending to do about it. I took a long, deep breath, sighed and then said "God! That poor poor girl." I thanked them for telling me so kindly, promised I was OK over and over and kept taking sharp deep breaths as I came to terms with it all. Slowly, ever so slowly, as the words "yes yes I'm fine, don't worry" kept coming out of my mouth, the impact of the news, the injustice, the recent pain I'd endured and finally the anger and frustration at how unfair the situation was, all started to erupt.

My eyes began leaking, no amount of wiping would stop the tears. My stomach lurched, my throat tightened and I was struggling to take in enough air to keep me from passing out.

It was just so wrong. Whoever was in charge had got it wrong. They'd put that baby in the wrong body!!! I'm over here! I'm ready, waiting, in fact I'm desperate. And yet, that baby would soon no longer be. Not planned, not wanted and soon not to be. It was an agony like no other. The pain mixed with anger was intense.

During the weeks that followed I helped support the girl, showed empathy, told her not to worry about my feelings. "I'm fine." I wasn't fine. It was a completely shitty scenario that nobody would have ever wished on either of us. In my then 38 years, I had never, (and still to this day as I write) ever experienced knowing anyone that had been through an abortion. Now, whilst desperate for a child, just a short time after an IVF cycle and lost pregnancy, here I was, supporting someone close to me.

The timing was the injustice really. It was cruel. It hurt like hell.

And, as with any grief or loss, the world around you simply carries on. That was how it felt at that time. I was stuck in a situation, couldn't move any which way to relieve the pain, and yet the rest of the world was carrying on, moving on and I felt left behind. I wanted to say to people "woohoo! I'm still here you know, still not pregnant, stuck in this infertile chapter" I wanted to shout out "Stop, stop, wait for me, don't carry on with your lives, I need to catch up!" Days and weeks passed and they were the days and weeks I was supposed to be getting more pregnant. We were flying through the calendar towards the end of the year and I was overwhelmed with all the events coming up that would now be different, as I wasn't going to be carrying my second child. The baby would have been born in July. Now, I wouldn't have a new baby for my whole family to coo over at my brother's wedding in September, Zac would definitely have started school before I had a baby, so I couldn't be on maternity leave and collect him each day and I now couldn't create a new bedroom for him as he may as well stay in the nursery that didn't have an impending new occupant. Time would continue to move on, events would come and go but my circumstances were still the same. It felt like I had fallen off the ride, like I had stalled and was stuck in a limbo whilst watching the world and everything around me move on without me. I broke my heart most days through December as the enormity of how different the following year was going to now be crushed my emotions.

As I walked round the shops Christmas shopping, the overwhelming feeling that I wasn't pregnant was almost too much to bear. From not having to carefully think about how heavy my bags where to every shop seeming to thrust 'Baby's First Christmas' items in my face. The reality really, really upset me. I knew it was partly because I was allowing the feelings to consume me, but they were so strong and I still felt so weak from the drugs and chest infection, that it was all too easy for the slightest thought to upset me. These were extremely sensitive weeks when the thoughts of not being able to have another baby were all consuming. I was literally on the brink of tears most of the time. Even writing Christmas cards was hard, as I had thought I might be writing to tell people we were expecting. Now I wasn't and it hurt. There would be no mention of Bump on our cards.

As it turned out, despite leaving arrangements to a last minute rush, Zac's birthday party was fantastic that year. In the end I couldn't find one pirate entertainer in East Yorkshire who was available that Sunday. I could get a Fireman which would have been great the previous year, but my soon to be

4 year old was now into Jake and the Neverland Pirates and Captain Hook. Fireman Sam was so last year! Daddy and Uncle Andrew came to the rescue however. We hired fabulous pirate costumes and they dressed up to entertain all the kids, hiding outside and peeking through windows, making them walk the cardboard plank and best of all, simply chasing them round the hall. I hadn't laughed so much in ages. They both really got into character and the kids loved it. I think the parents perhaps loved it more and many of them said it was the best entertainment they had seen in ages. Zac's little friend Lydia needed a little reassurance that Captain Swashbuckle was in fact Zac's daddy, so Zac took her up and whispered, "Is that really you daddy? It is isn't it?" It was so cute and he was so proud!

He seemed to be growing up so fast at that time and his development was coming on leaps and bounds. He was growing in confidence, his speech was improving and you could see that he and his friends were starting to form their own amusement with each other and needing their parents to entertain them less and less. Time seemed to be flying when I looked at how all of them were growing up.

A few days later, we were over at Mums for Christmas. By this time I was still under the weather and that day, I didn't really feel myself but put it down to the stress of wrapping and packing everything to go to my Mums. As we had done for many years, Mum and I were planning on going to Christmas Eve Midnight Mass, and Jason was going to stay at home to look after Zac. As we got ready to leave, I quickly nipped upstairs to the toilet and got the shock of my life. My period had arrived. That explained why I felt so rough. It was a real slap in the face. I sat for a short time on the toilet and just cried. This was the first period since the loss and a stark reminder that I definitely wasn't pregnant. I felt really flat.

During Mass I sang my heart out to all the carols. I felt the words wash through me and suddenly felt warm and comforted that perhaps the baby was going to come to me after all. "Glory to the newborn king", "Oh come let us adore him" and "Yet in thy dark streets shineth, the everlasting light, the hopes and fears of all the years, are met in thee tonight". I had always loved singing and it always made me feel good, but that night, listening to so many songs about the celebration of a new baby seemed to lift my spirits once more and was a huge tonic.

As expected Christmas Day was lovely but again, also hard in some ways. We are blessed with a loving family and we have always made a big fuss at birthdays and Christmas and this year was no exception. Zac was overjoyed that Santa had found him at Grandma's house and overjoyed at his huge pirate ship and electric guitar. He was amazed, if not perhaps slightly frightened, when he saw a bite out of the mince pie and found one of the reindeers' bells on the patio where their food had been. He was so grown up in some ways but still our cute baby boy in others. We hadn't really thought about how scary it could be to a four year old to see 'proof' that a strange man had been downstairs and a load of reindeer in the garden, whilst he slept upstairs!!

As much as I enjoyed the feasting and presents I still felt slightly distant from the celebrations and couldn't help but wonder how different it would have been if we'd been successful. I constantly tried to shake the thoughts from my head but they seemed ever-present and all consuming. My heart melted when I saw Zac with both Minnie and Zara, playing with them, showing them how their presents worked and couldn't help but think about how different the following Christmas would have been, had this last cycle been successful. Next Christmas we would have had a baby to buy for, but now that dream was gone. And yet, after starting my period, which had made me feel better and then singing my heart out in church, I was still thoughtful but perhaps my feelings were a little less desolate.

We began thinking more and more clearly as the days passed across the Christmas holidays and Jason and I spent some time together. My chest infection had started to lift a little and with the emotional cloud lifting from our hearts also, we started to rationalise recent events. Was it ever probable that I would have ever gotten pregnant given all that was stacked against me at that time? I was really poorly with the hyper stimulation, I had a chest infection and an ear infection and with all that combined, I was a physical and emotional wreck. With the emotional side of the recent rollercoaster, trying to manage my feelings around others, control my feelings and symptoms around Zac, whilst having my mind play tricks on me about possible outcomes, was it really any wonder I miscarried? I was confident that it was a simple case of primeval 'fight or flight' in action and that at that moment, my body was telling itself that it was not fit enough to have an additional life drain it further and therefore rejected that life. I was not a safe haven to nurture an embryo and so that life did not proceed. It made sense, gave me some rationality to the situation and made me more determined to learn from the first attempt to ensure the second would work.

Many a time through the treatment I'd said "never again" after experiencing how bad it could be, but now it was all I wanted to do. I couldn't wait to go again. Despair was starting to make way for hope and optimism and as much as the world was carrying on, I was now more than ready to get back on the ride.

Every time I'd watch Zac with his favourite Fireman Sam figures I'd imagine what it would be like for him playing with a younger brother or sister. Would he share, would the baby even like Fireman Sam, or might it be a little sister who preferred fairies and princesses and insisted Zac play with her toys? Sometimes my mind would just wander imagining what life could be like if we tried again and were successful.

Would Zac shoot goals and the little one be keeper? Would they share a bath or would Zac then be of an age that he'd be too shy? Would they play, play fight or just fight? Would they even be alike or would the new baby be a completely different child to Zac? A thousand and one questions used to fill my mind and it was as exciting as it was frustrating not to be in control of the answers.

On the first work day after the Christmas break, I called Roxanne at the clinic to report the date of my period and tell them I wanted to try again. I told her I had really missed them and she was quick to say, "We've missed you too!" She made me smile, I felt immediately that I was back on it, part of the gang again and we were off and running with our second attempt!

Back on it

I went back to the clinic for our first appointment where I was to meet the team, talk through the last cycle and decide on our new plan. As we had frozen three embryos from the last round, we were going to use them for this cycle, which would mean I wouldn't have to go through the stimulation drugs. It felt right and positive that it had worked out this way and I felt that perhaps I shouldn't be disappointed in the first cycle not working, as this was always how it was meant to be. I would be well this time when they did the transfer and therefore, hopefully have a better chance of keeping the embryo.

As the meeting was simply to go through the plan that we had previously discussed with them, Jason and I agreed that I would go on my own. I was excited but as I drove nearer to the hospital I became overwhelmingly anxious. I could feel my eyes start to tear up and I called Jason to admit that I was so desperate to get into the clinic, to be near the laboratory and be near our embryos again. I longed to be near them and as I got closer, I began to realise just how much I had been thinking about them and how much I loved them already. They were just a few cells each, but they were mine and could be my babies. I just wanted to be under the same roof as them so badly I felt I could burst. He reassured me that I didn't sound daft. They might grow to be Zac's brother or sister. In fact, at one time Zac had been just a few cells inside me and now he was our precious boy. Some people view embryos differently, but in my eyes, they were mine and Jason's offspring.

I met some of the nurses in the reception area and as usual they made me extremely welcome with their warmth and kindness. As I was left alone, I cried softly in the waiting area, wiping away slow tear after slow tear; a mixture of being suddenly flung back into this world again and being just two rooms away from our embys. It felt great to be back, to talk to the nurses and I felt hugely positive, but the emotions were overwhelming.

I was shown into one of the consultation rooms where Debbie was to talk through the next steps. It was lovely to see her again, she always made me laugh and I really felt comfortable talking to her. We talked about the drugs and the differences between a fresh and frozen cycle. It all began to feel quite exciting again.

However, neither Jason nor I had realised that we would need to decide that day, how many of our three frozen embryos we wanted to defrost.

Debbie talked me through the pros and cons and I listened intently but couldn't focus or make a decision. I knew they were just embryos, just cells but despite being so small they were all so important to me, all three of them. I felt like they were asking me to choose between them. I felt like they had feelings, a soul and I could never leave one behind but knew they would never transfer three. What if I was successful after transferring two embryos and had twins, what would happen to the last one? I knew right there and then I could never destroy it or leave it frozen, I would have to come back and get it and create its life.

I know some people see this stage very differently and probably think me daft for having such thoughts but that was how I felt about them. They were mine, part of our family whatever stage they were at and I could never destroy them. I felt such a strong love and protective feeling towards them in both my head and my heart and I knew I could never leave nor destroy them. There was of course the chance that none of them would survive the freeze and defrost process and we may not be able to proceed at all, but if that happened it seemed that fate had decided rather than the weight of that decision on my sensitive shoulders.

I guess it was inevitable that it would happen, but I started to cry, to weep again. Already, I was just hours into the new cycle and I was crying. I simply hadn't expected to have to make this decision today and Jason and I hadn't even discussed it together. The weight of the implications was huge and the thought that at some point I would have to destroy one was incredibly painful.

Earlier I'd been giddy with Debbie at the thought that with the frozen cycle they would transfer two embryos. For some bizarre reason I had long thought it was my destiny that I would have twins and I felt a flurry of excitement at the prospect that it was simply meant to turn out like that with this second, frozen cycle. There were many reasons why I thought I might have twins, and none of them to do with genetics, but latterly Zac had been insistent that he wanted a boy baby and a girl baby, two not one, which had only sought to compound my belief that it was meant to be that I should have two together. I mentioned this to Debbie who did a wonderful job at finding a balance of remaining professional by saying "well you never know" but also being giddy with me. I needed to be excited but I knew she also needed to keep me grounded. She didn't make me feel silly at talking about what I thought was my destiny but she did ensure my feet stayed firmly on the ground.

As I had mentioned Zac's thoughts on another baby, she asked me about him. As ever, I over enthused about my gorgeous boy and got my phone out to proudly show her photos. I loved showing him off and always felt immensely proud as I gushed over the latest funny stories. And then I stopped. Suddenly I felt shame and embarrassment.

All of a sudden, telling the clinic I already had a little boy felt wrong. Like it was a secret I should keep to myself. I had always talked to them about my longing for a baby and yet all along I had one at home. They meet couples every day longing for a child, many of whom, despite the best treatment, will never be a parent. Yet here I was, crying about my next cycle of treatment, when already I had what so many of them longed for.

Would Debbie look at me any differently now knowing I had a child? Would she wonder why I was here in the clinic and would she think I was being greedy at going through so much treatment when I was lucky enough to already have a child? Suddenly talking about Zac, my child, my boy, seemed hard to do with her. Saying I had a child seemed to be a sort of cheat, a shameful admission. For some reason I felt I needed to say that we had been given Clomid from this very clinic to have Zac, so it was OK for them to know that we had him. I was almost justifying my pursuit of others by the fact that it had been difficult to have my first for some reason.

At that moment I didn't think that the team met all sorts of couple from all sorts of backgrounds, all with different situations and reasons for wanting IVF treatment. You could have a house full of children but if you still wanted another and were struggling to conceive, this was simply a route to help you. You didn't have to be without a child to want or need IVF and in my saner moments I really knew this, but at that time, for some reason I felt that I shouldn't be there. I felt guilty for taking up their time.

After much chat and consideration of our options I decided that Mother Nature always had the final say anyway and therefore the sensible thing was to defrost all three frozen embryos and go with the two embryos that survived the aggressive defrosting process the best and that ultimately had the best chance of survival. This felt a comfortable decision and one that I felt I could live with for the rest of my days, but having said that, before finally confirming I asked to check with Jason that he agreed. Fortunately he did. The thought of being successful and feeling that our family was complete and then at a later date having to decide that the last one in the lab should be destroyed, was simply too much too bear and something I never ever wanted to have to do. Neither did I ever feel that I could donate any. I felt so connected to them, that they were my children, my bloodline and I was their Mummy. I admire those who do donate eggs, sperm or embryos so much, they give others the chance of a family and for that I wholeheartedly applaud them. Perhaps I applaud them more because I know it is not something I could do. After what we have been through, I view things slightly differently, which is why what they do is so terrifically special.

I took my appointment card, waited for my invoice, sent off my cheque and arranged to collect the drugs a couple of days later. We were off!

It felt strange but great to be starting again. I had learned at lot from the first cycle and felt more comfortable than I had done previously. I began to read up on the treatment and complimentary treatments. I often laughed at just how different men and women can be at times, but in this instance put it down to it purely being my body that was undergoing the invasive treatment rather than Jason's that meant I was driving forward, making appointments, reading books and surfing the internet. Every so often he would ask me a question and sometimes I would simply answer him giving him all the details but at other times I would get cross that he expected me to know the answer or to find out and that he hadn't investigated anything for himself. I was being grossly unfair on him but sometimes his questions about information that I had taken the trouble to research would frustrate me. Other times, he'd make me laugh and I'd reply, "It's a bloody good job I know about that isn't it?"

I dabbled with the infertility websites and forums once more but again; it all just made me feel sad. My recent experience was too raw and now on my next cycle, I simply wasn't in a position to invite further sadness. There was no place for negativity in my life at that time. Once more, I didn't feel it was a club I did or wanted to belong to. Perhaps this was denial, but it felt like a world full of strangers in desperate but different circumstances to me. I wanted to be optimistic that I was going to come out with a positive result this time and didn't want or need any negative persuasion that this may not be the case. Failure was an option, a reality I knew that, but I wasn't about to make it a consideration right now. I didn't go onto another forum after that.

I was however enlightened by a book. I bought a guide to IVF by a London based fertility expert and when it arrived it was the size of a bible. I was working my way through it when one paragraph struck me and really connected with me. It was very short but it discussed the misplaced guilt existing parents feel when wanting another child yet struggle and require IVF. It discussed how they often met people who had children who felt they were already so lucky and felt guilty at wanting more. They then went on to discuss that this should not be the case and that one shouldn't feel guilty at all, indeed having children already can often be the trigger to make you want more, to provide a sibling. That was me! They were completely describing me, my situation and my feelings. I did feel guilty, I was driven by a natural desire for more children but I was also driven by Zac. It was almost therapeutic to think that it really was OK to want another child and that I should try to shake off any guilt if it surfaced again. It was a very useful paragraph in what was otherwise a very complex book! I would later learn, that this enlightenment and realisation that there was far too little attention paid to this condition, was in fact the very first spark that led to my mission to raise the profile of Secondary Infertility.

Whilst still excited about being on our journey to having another child again, there was many a moment when we did question what on earth we were thinking. We took Zac's friends Harry and Eva out for the day to the local soft play centre and then to McDonalds where all three ran about, screamed and giggled between themselves. Taking three kids out was so different to just a day out with Zac and their excitement made them almost uncontrollable. It was utter chaos and Jason and I would look between each other and laugh saying: "We want more kids?" We kept cracking up laughing as we saw, what we hoped was our future, playing out in front of us and as we mopped up coke and asked them to keep the noise down for the tenth time, it all looked and felt very stressful!

On another occasion, Zac was poorly and cried nearly all night. I had changed the bed twice already and we had towels everywhere, all over the floor. Jason and I both had early meetings the next day but didn't get a wink of sleep as our tired, cranky little boy wailed through every hour. What if we had to look after another one? What if he woke the other one up too? What if both kids were ill at the same time? Could we both work if we had two poorly children up all night? What were we doing?

Work continued to be my safe haven. I was busy business planning for the forthcoming year with Dom and Emma, which was exciting as we were building a strong blueprint to move us forward into a new area of business and strengthen up existing services. There was a real sense of optimism and positivity throughout the whole team, we were all really going for it. It was a great feeling but I couldn't help but feel frustrated that I was still there planning for the business. I wanted to be planning my family. This wasn't the path I thought I was going to be taking, not the one I really wanted to be on. I thrived off planning for the agency and was excited about our plans for growth but at the same time, with each meeting, I grew internally angry that I was focussing on this area. It wasn't meant to be like this.

Round 2

As round two progressed, I felt really well in myself and really optimistic. As we had decided to defrost three and progress with the two strongest embryos my mind was consumed with two of everything. Car seats, needing a new car, their clothes, would I want two the same gender or one of each? Having always had a feeling I'd have twins and now, with a real chance in having two embryos put back, I was feeling that fate was about to be sealed. One day as we sat having lunch in the office, we were discussing the treatment and Emma mentioned that she thought I was going to have two. She reeled in shock when I agreed, replying: "Yes, so do I!"

As retrieval day grew closer I planned my absence with work better. We started handovers earlier and learning lessons from last time, I let the girls take over more instead of retaining much of the work myself, which turned out to be too stressful for everyone. The whole office knew what was going on but it was fairly unspoken and I was grateful for this discretion. The girls who were our account managers took more of the strain of the accounts and it was February, which turned out to be a much quieter period to take off than November so it was altogether a lot less stressful. I even took the day before off to relax at home, which I hadn't done the last time. I kept Zac off nursery with me to have a bit of quality mummy time, which was lovely. I knew that if we were to be successful, the following day would be the start of many more months of pain, swelling and ultimately too little time to spend with him whilst feeling well, so I relished every second we could enjoy together.

On the day of retrieval we were expecting a call from the clinic, between 9.30 and 11am, advising us whether or not the embryos had survived the defrost. After taking Zac to nursery, I came home and tried to keep myself busy whilst trying to work out our chances of any surviving. Apparently the defrosting was an aggressive process and there was no guarantee this cycle would progress any further.

At 9.55am, the call came. Two out of the three embryos had survived! The embryologist asked what time could we come in and I made her laugh by instantly replying, "now?" They asked us not to rush and said they would see us at 11.15am.

They'd survived!

I broke down crying as I put the phone down. They had overcome their final hurdle. They had been strong enough to survive; our little embryos had made it through. The last hurdle was beyond my control and I'd bottled up the anxiety about whether or not we would be successful, to such a degree that my body now shook with the relief that they'd survived and we were on! Jason once again held me in his arms in our bedroom doorway, as I relieved some tension through sobbing, but we were quick to head into the bedroom and get changed to go.

Once again I dressed smartly. I felt like I wanted to be a mum that they could be proud of, so wore my new jeans, white shirt, new black stilettos and lovely fitted grey, wool coat. Ridiculous I know. As if what I wore mattered to anyone or made a difference to the outcome, but it really helped me and I felt excited as we set off.

It was really great seeing the team again as they busied themselves round the clinic and welcomed us into the bay for me to change. I was really excited as we confirmed our names and details and it was confirmed again that we were to have two embryos transferred.

One was grade 2 out of 3 and one was 1.5, but they were happy with the quality of both of them so were happy to transfer them both.

The procedure took much longer this time, 40 minutes in total. I was on the bed with my legs in stirrups all that time whilst Denise tried over and again to get the catheter inserted into the correct place in my cervix. My kink was severe this time and despite trying the softer instrument it still wouldn't find it's way to the correct position. The embryos were taken back into the lab into the warmth of the 'incubator'. I felt frustrated that they wouldn't go in and felt I was letting them down. I was desperate to get them inside me, longed for them and worried for their survival, but we were assured that they would be OK there for the time being. I could feel big, fat, warm tears roll down my cheeks as they were taken back to the lab, I wanted to tell them I was so, so sorry for the messing round and I started to think the worst about this cycle and my prospects of being a mum to the two of them. I was falling at this hurdle and they weren't even inside me! What was wrong with me? I was reassured by Jason and the team and realised I needed to get a grip, remain calm and start to try to relax.

Each time they tried I got a real intense acute pain as they pushed the catheter. After several attempts, Denise called Professor Killick to come and take a look and have a try. Whilst the team involved were always lovely and I trusted them implicitly, it was also nice to have Prof involved and again, I felt like it was fate. That he was going to do the transfer was some sort of positive omen about this attempt.

In his usual, crazy demeanour he began waffling on to try to distract and relax me and as usual, he made me giggle. He was telling us a story about how he once had a patient who was a dentist who advised him that they relaxed patients with a mirror on the ceiling but that he didn't think that was appropriate for clients in his line of work and asked me what did I think? He was just hysterical and despite still having my legs in stirrups, I was laughing my head off by now. He had just finished getting his gloves on and putting the seat to the right height when a horrendous terrifying alarm went off. It was so loud and frightening I jumped out of my skin and immediately thought the worst. Was there a problem with the equipment, or worse still, me? It was his mobile ringtone. It was on the setting of a ship's horn that went off on the highest volume setting repeatedly, which, he later explained, was to ensure he heard it! He then went on to answer the call and talk to the caller about where he was, what he was doing and how he'd meet them in Ultrasound in 10 minutes! Incredible! We were all laughing our heads off and I was by this stage under such strain that my emotions needed a valve from which to escape and for once it was through laughter rather than tears. I was hysterical. I simply could not stop laughing at him! The terrifying thought that an alarm was going off in theatre only for it to be his mobile, and then for him to have a full on conversation whilst I'm laid there with my legs in the air waiting for him to finish, was just too funny. I was shaking uncontrollably and there were tears and snot all over my face that Jason had to keep wiping away for me! Every time I took a deep breath to try to compose myself, I'd crack up laughing again and of course we couldn't proceed until I could keep still. The team were so patient but it took the best part of 10 minutes for me to calm down and compose myself!

The team decided to internally anaesthetise my cervix in several places so that they could use more force to push the catheter past the kinks. I couldn't feel a thing, felt more relaxed and eventually they successfully transferred both embryos. We saw two tiny white 'stars' in my uterus on the scan and everyone was happy that the transfer had gone well. Including Prof, who was by now putting his jacket on and was on his way to Ultrasound!

The two week wait – take two!

I was anxious of course, but second time round I was really excited. Having gone through the treatment once before I felt more relaxed in the comfort of understanding the process and what to expect. It was however, an extremely long two weeks to wait. It definitely seemed longer than last time. I felt really well in myself and I think that made time drag all the more as I was more alert and aware of time and what was happening, without a chest infection or any side affects of the drugs to distract me. We slowly slipped back into normality and I went back to work where every hour really dragged. It was the time of year of our company's anniversary again and like every year, we had arranged a meal out for Dom, Emma and myself and our partners to celebrate. We had had the date booked for sometime but as bad luck would have it, it happened to be booked for the night of the day I was due to take the pregnancy test. A friend suggested I get the meal moved but as it was so hard to juggle everyone's diaries and the timing was perfect for our anniversary, I took some persuading. I didn't want to fuss or make a point of the events of the day but at the same time, irrespective of the result, going out for dinner that night was not the best idea, so in the end we postponed the meal until the following week.

This time we had told hardly anybody we were doing the treatment. People were used to me not drinking now so it didn't raise any suspicions when we went out and I was drinking coke. We went out to celebrate a friend's birthday the weekend before the test and I was struggling to find something to wear. I hadn't really been stressed about what to wear in the days running up to the night out, as I knew I had 2 new dresses I'd not worn before, so there wasn't the usual flapping about my wardrobe. That night though when I was getting ready, my boobs were suddenly far too huge to fit into one of the dresses and they simply overflowed in the other, making me look like some sort of cheap call girl. In the end I opted for a dress they'd all seen before and whilst my boobs still looked enormous they didn't look like they needed a place setting of their own! I didn't really care what I was wearing that night and I felt in great spirits. I felt pregnant, I looked pregnant and I was hopefully days away from confirming that I was.

Half way through the night, I went to the Ladies with one of my girlfriends and told her I was excited that I was about to find out later that week. She was shocked that she didn't know how far on we were with the treatment but said she understood why we had kept it to ourselves. Talking about it made it seem all the more real and walking back to the table, the rest of the party could be forgiven for thinking I was drunk as I was giggly with a huge smile on my face. I loved finally talking about it and I just loved sitting amongst my friends feeling so positively pregnant after all this time.

As the week went on I got more and more tired. I literally felt like lying down in the office at times and from the moment I walked in the house each evening I couldn't wait to get to bed. I kept remembering my Mum's words when I was pregnant with Zac and first complaining about being so tired when she said: "your body is creating a baby in there, you're bound to be tired!" It made me excited to remember, to think about everything that was going on inside me and perhaps this time, I was growing two babies so of course I was definitely going to feel really tired!

I was also increasingly nauseous. The first time I got a flurry was really strange and I daren't really acknowledge it. Was that morning sickness really? The second then third times, I knew there was no mistaking that familiar feeling and despite the queasiness, I was thrilled each time a wave came over me. It was happening more and more often and stronger each time. Three days before I was due to take the test, I opened the dishwasher and the smell just hit my stomach making me lurch for the downstairs toilet. I just made it in time. This was definitely morning sickness and the familiar feeling made me almost shudder with excitement. I was sick pretty much every day of my pregnancy with Zac and most days, would vomit 6 or 7 times from the moment I woke up. I carried sick bowls in the car for any length of journey and often had to literally run out of meetings to get to the toilet. To have the symptoms so severe, I was more than familiar with the particular type of nausea and whilst I wasn't looking forward to the prospect of vomiting day in, day out, I was beyond excited that this was definitely a sure sign of a new pregnancy.

I knew I was walking round smiling all the time. When I was in the house, I was permanently consumed with the thought that I had my babies inside me. I embraced Zac whenever I could get hold of him and kept hold of him just that little bit longer. Would we have another Zac? Could we possibly create another child as wonderful as our first? I simply couldn't wait to find out and I was thrilled at the prospect of introducing him to his new sibling or siblings! The thought of twin babies was nothing short of exciting. I wasn't in any place to dwell on the potential dangers or downsides of having two babies and I'm sure any thought of what life might be like in the future must have made me glow on the outside, reflecting just how giddy I was on the inside.

I felt pregnant. The feeling was overwhelming. The excitement was all consuming. I'm not a betting person but I would have bet my mortgage in those days that there was not a chance I couldn't be pregnant. As each day passed I became more and more convinced that I was definitely carrying one if not two babies.

During one of our office chats Emma confirmed that she thought I was pregnant too. She said I just looked pregnant and that my boobs were enormous and round! It was true, my boobs had grown, I'd lost my waist, another symptom that I had with Zac and I had a real glow about me.

I walked round as if it had already been confirmed. Being pregnant consumed all my thoughts and all my daydreaming was about positive baby thoughts and how exciting the next few months were going to be. That said, whenever I spoke about it to anyone else, I always said that whilst I felt pregnant, it could just be the drugs giving me the symptoms. I had been warned that the drugs were designed to tell your body you were pregnant so that the uterus wouldn't shed the wall lining and would retain the embryos, so I knew that all these symptoms could simply be as a result of this particular set of drugs. I knew this could be the explanation, but I didn't believe it. I heard myself telling people, I kept telling myself in fact and I had heard it with my own ears from the clinic, but now, with such strong symptoms, in my heart of heart, I was convinced that there was no other possible explanation other than pregnancy. The symptoms were so strong, so similar to how I was when pregnant with Zac. I just felt pregnant.

I was due to take the pregnancy test on the Friday and as the week went on, I strangely became more and more relaxed as the symptoms persisted and if anything became stronger. Whilst serving dinner on the Thursday evening, I had to drop everything and run to the toilet where I vomited for about 5 minutes. Zac was asking if I was all right and Jason was sat at the dinner table looking spooked. I walked back in, reassured Zac that mummy was fine and looked over to Jason who had a strange mix of delight and fear across his face as the reality of what it could mean really dawned on him.

After dinner, when neither of us had obviously mentioned what had happened for fear of worrying or troubling Zac, we sat back and simply looked at each other. I couldn't help but smirk, I knew I was smirking but I didn't know what to say, I couldn't find any words. Jason was starting to list all the examples of symptoms that had become more obvious and frequent over the past few days and I heard myself trying to put it all into perspective for him so he didn't get carried away. I was explaining to him again that the clinic had said it could be the drugs in a way that made out I thought he was being ridiculous and should be more cautious, when in fact, I felt exactly the same! Quickly though, he switched his views as well and began explaining each example away that it was probably the effect of the drugs, in a way trying to keep both of us and our excitement in check. Yet we just kept looking at each other, neither wanting to get too giddy, but at the same time, both wanting to explode as the possibilities started to feel so real.

Finally, I said: "I'm not sure I should say this, but I really don't think I need to do the test tomorrow. I really feel really pregnant. I am convinced I am."

Of course we were going to the do the test the next day anyway and that night as I got ready for bed, I felt a strange mix of excitement and anxiety. I couldn't wait for the morning but I had also enjoyed that last week feeling so pregnant that the thought that there was a chance I might not be, so that the feeling might end, was absolutely terrifying. I didn't want it to end. I had loved that week so much. Loved being sick even! Tomorrow would be a game changer either way. It wouldn't be life as we knew it whatever the outcome. If the result was positive, that would throw us into the world of babies again and that would be terribly exciting but if by any slight chance the result was going to be negative, this lovely warm feeling of being pregnant would end and we'd be flung straight back into the painful world of infertility and wondering where our life would end up. That slight chance of that negative result added to my nausea that night.

The wait was over

We both awoke early, before Zac, which was unusual but it felt so right, almost as if he knew we needed some time on our own that morning. As soon as we roused, we both went to the ensuite and I peed on two sticks, the one from the hospital and a digital one from the chemist. Once more I stayed in the bathroom and waited for the result and Jason busied himself in the bedroom. I felt strangely calm and, more than ever before, I simply felt it was agonising waiting for the result. I couldn't wait to see the smiley face. I was desperate to leap into Jason's arms to hug him, squeeze him, cry, laugh and celebrate our impending new baby or babies. The excitement was almost unbearable. My mouth was dry and although my tummy was swollen, I could feel that it was also in knots as we waited.

It wouldn't be an understatement to say I literally leapt back away from the sticks. My gasp was so loud that Jason jumped. There was no other sound, no words, just silence as I held the sticks with one hand and put the other hand to my mouth. Negative. Both sticks showed negative.

It couldn't be. They must be wrong. They must both be wrong, both be faulty. Or the date must be wrong and it was too soon to do the test. It just couldn't be negative.

Sadly of course, they weren't wrong and as I continued to stand there staring in disbelief at both sticks, the hospital indicator was clearly getting stronger and stronger, confirming that there was no pregnancy, no baby, no happy ending.

I was stunned. Totally shocked by the result. I had always said it could have been the drugs giving me the symptoms but I had never really believed it. They were so strong, so frequent, so like my last pregnancy with Zac, that every part of my body believed I was definitely pregnant. I kept asking myself "How could I not be pregnant".

It felt as if the pregnancy had been taken away from me. That morning someone took my future away from me. It felt like I had been on a track for sure and now, I had been unceremoniously thrown off it, not allowed to go any further. The end of the road. You've had two weeks to enjoy it, now get off the ride!

I still felt sick, my boobs were enormous and sore, my sides had thickened and I just felt so pregnant. And yet, I had to try to get my head around the result and start to believe that I wasn't.

I wanted to do another test immediately, as I couldn't get passed the thought that they must have been faulty, but Jason told me not to do another, don't waste a test or upset myself further. Clearly it was conclusive. Clearly it wasn't a faulty test. There was no baby.

I didn't cry. I was numb. Jason had a small cry but I was almost paralysed. I couldn't go to him, couldn't hug him, I simply couldn't move. The result wouldn't sink in, it was as if my body was in limbo and before it could react I had to believe what the result was telling me. Jason went into the bedroom but my feet were rooted to the soft mat in the bathroom. I just kept looking at the sticks. It wasn't supposed to be like this.

I wasn't bleeding like last time, I hadn't even had a show and I felt fit and well and happy and…yet none of that mattered. I wasn't pregnant. I had never been pregnant this time. It just hadn't worked.

Zac woke and cried out for me, so I grabbed my dressing down and brought him downstairs for breakfast. Somehow a child's cry and Mother Nature can suddenly make you function and jump into action, whether it is in the dead of night or in a moment of utter sorrow. I found myself carrying him, making him comfortable on the sofa, turning on the TV for him and then sitting in silence next to him. I didn't hold him or cuddle him; I just sat closely next to him. I couldn't bear for him to sense anything was wrong, I didn't have the words of comfort or explanation for him just yet. I needed him to remain ignorant to what was going on for now and I knew I couldn't be strong if he should start with his usual inquisitiveness.

Jason came down shortly after and turned the kettle on. He asked if I was all right and I just nodded and said yes. I was surprised to hear myself say yes, but at that moment I did feel all right. It hadn't really sunk in and I couldn't get my head around what had happened, so actually I did feel OK. I didn't feel sad, didn't feel heartbroken and didn't feel like tears were going to come at all.

I was remarkably OK, yes. I looked across at my sorrowful husband, busying himself in the kitchen getting his breakfast and making us cups of tea. Part of me felt compelled to go and hug and comfort him, but a larger part of me sensed that right now, that wasn't going to help either of us, especially with Zac in the room.

It was nearly 8am and I knew my Mum would be pacing the floor but I just didn't want to speak to anyone, not even her. I couldn't face calling, didn't know what to say really and certainly didn't want to have a full-blown discussion about it.

I texted her. I wanted her to stop worrying but equally couldn't face the reality of saying the words, so I just wrote: 'I'm not pregnant. Two tests so it's deffo x so shocked I'll call later xx'

Quarter of an hour later I was still sat in the same place on the sofa and was now stroking Zac's head. My whole world was turned upside down, it was like I'd fallen off a fairground ride and couldn't get back on. And now feeling his warmth against me I felt that I had let Zac down as well. I was supposed to be telling him in a few weeks that he was going to have a baby brother or sister, or both, and the thought that that conversation wasn't now going to happen was the catalyst that made my body finally realise, accept and deal with the reality that this cycle was over.

Tears started to form and I tried to wipe them. My eyes were stinging and I could sense that my body was starting to react to the news. Shock was making way for grief and I had no idea how to stop the emotion so I sent Zac upstairs to choose his clothes for the day and Jason came over and pulled me up into his arms. The tears started to come and my body started to shake. A desperate sobbing in response to the total disbelief at what had actually caused these tears. It felt good to be in Jason's arms, to hold him too, but suddenly a huge painful wave came over me at the added pain I must have caused him after what I'd said to him the night before. I told him I was so, so sorry for what I had said at the dinner table. I should never have said I thought I was pregnant and to do so, I really felt was cruel to him. It was heartbreaking enough for me, but to think that I had said that to him, when he was wasn't in control of the feelings in the body creating and carrying the child, was overwhelmingly painful for me. I was convinced enough I was pregnant that he should believe me and I truly regretted ever saying anything to him. I felt a huge burden at his pain, the pain I had helped cause. Of course he reassured me that he too had been convinced that I was, but that didn't ease my guilt at saying those words. I had been wrong to say that to him and bitterly regretted it, which only added to the hurt that morning.

I texted the few friends that knew about the treatment, but felt at a loss to know what to say. When their words of comfort and friendship came back I repeatedly just texted 'I know it's shit, it's just shit', which is exactly how I felt but moreover it was a signal that I didn't want to discuss it any more with anyone. There was nothing anyone could do or say to change the result or take the pain away, so I wanted to avoid all conversation completely.

I dropped Zac off at nursery and despite the bit of make up I'd slapped on, I looked simply dreadful and as the usually cheery Sam opened the door to welcome Zac in, she automatically did a double take and asked if I was OK. I nodded, half smiled and just said "yes thanks" as I busied myself helping Zac take this shoes off and get his slippers on. I kissed him and held him long and hard. Letting go of him that morning was so hard but I knew I had to before I broke down. Sam had noticed and caught my eye as I stood up. I had no idea if she knew we'd been trying or having treatment but heard myself say: "Another round of IVF hasn't worked". I could feel hot, wet tears slowly run down each cheek. She put her arm round me and rubbed my own arm, said she was so sorry and taking a deep breath, I shook off the tears and made my way out. I don't know why I told her other than perhaps I thought she might think it was something more serious. More serious? Well with perspective, nobody had died at least and I didn't want to cause undue alarm. Saying the words made the shock and truth sink in a little deeper. It really hurt.

This time hit me much worse than the first time. I felt angry more quickly. I could feel the anger through my limbs, my stiff arms and clenched fists and I'm sure if I'd left the house, I could easily have punched something or someone. It was more than not being pregnant this time, I literally felt bereft, like someone had taken a pregnancy away from me. Last time I had been pregnant but never really believed it as I'd been so poorly and been bleeding and yet despite obviously never being pregnant at all this time, the pain was a hundred times more intense, because I thought I was.

I had to ring the clinic in the afternoon to tell them the result. My voice broke as I said the words 'the tests were negative'. Yet again they were sympathetic, saying they were so sorry and that they would have an audit meeting to look at possible reasons why and then they would be in touch. And then it was over. Finished. Ended.

I felt cut loose, in freefall. There was no longer a track, no plan, and no baby. The clinic told me to stop taking the drugs immediately, but now I didn't want to, I wanted to keep taking them. They were part of being on this journey and I didn't want it to end.

Once the crying came it wouldn't stop. As the reality slowly began sinking in fully, the enormity of what it meant, reduced me to a sobbing wreck. I beat my fists on our coffee table. I found myself screaming out loud which broke down into a repetition of "No, No, No". Then I cried some more and roared in pain, as loud as I could and again reduced to sobbing "No, No" over and over again. I was clenching my teeth and throwing my head back whilst this curdling, growling sound came out of my throat and then yet again, as my neck tensed and jaw thrust forward, an awful scream came rushing out of me. I had never made such noises in my life and would have perhaps been a little shocked at my outbursts, had I not been so distraught. Tears, snot and saliva were pumping out of me, smeared all over my face and sometimes not wiped or bothered about at all. My head was starting to pound and I rubbed my hands firmly across and around my face, almost searching for an answer as to why this was happening. My hair was all over the place, as I repeatedly rubbed my hands backwards and forwards in frustration then tried to run my fingers through it, but resorting to roughly tying it back out of the way.

Perhaps it is a primeval way of letting out anger and pain, but the screaming and roaring was something that was happening involuntary and whilst it didn't take the hurt away, it did tire me out quickly which brought the screaming and shouting to an abrupt end. What was left was what felt like the broken shell of a girl. I had no emotion left inside me. I was exhausted and wrung out as I curled up on the floor, with a blanket wrapped round me, tucked between the coffee table and the sofa.

Occasionally I got up to get a drink or go to the toilet, but for most of the day, I sat or lay on the floor, weeping, wrapped in the blanket. I had known the day before that the chance of a negative result would be shattering, but I had never expected a reaction like this. I struggled to calm myself down, to be rational or to think clearly. I really felt like I was losing control of my emotions and my ability to deal with the situation. What I hadn't realised was that I simply needed to hit rock bottom with my grief and to let out all the pent up pain, before I could begin to start to deal with anything. It was probably quite good to have had that insane reaction, as strange and as scary as it was at the time.

Trying to cope moving on

I kept my head down all weekend and we stayed at home keeping ourselves busy and spending time with Zac. I received some really lovely, supportive messages from friends and whilst it was nice to receive them they just made me feel so utterly sad that we should be in that situation.

I went back to work on the Monday morning as normal. As I always dropped Zac at nursery first thing, I texted Emma to say she could tell the team before I arrived if she felt it was right to do so, but that I didn't want to talk about it with anyone. I walked into our office and without looking at her, said "don't ask me as I'm not ready to talk" and she knowingly started to distract us both with updates on current client projects. Hard as it was to concentrate or care at that moment it was a refreshing conversation that started to help me put the pieces back together.

The usual Monday morning team meeting started at 10am and amazingly I managed to get through it, contributing normally and was cheered by the thought that I seemed to be managing to function fine after all. Straight after the meeting, Emma asked if I wanted an update and after making a cup of tea, we returned back to the meeting room where I was determined not to think about the previous week. I told myself that there could be no discussion whatsoever as there could only be two scenarios, coping with the situation or not coping with the situation. There was no middle ground and I knew there would be no sniffle or small weep. If I thought about it and acknowledged the pain and grief I was struggling to smother, there would be no holding back, it would all come flooding out and this was no time and no place for that to happen.

She looked at me and hugged me. I broke down and I sobbed!

I should have known it would be impossible to hold back. I simply couldn't believe I was back at work and not pregnant. It wasn't meant to be like this. On Thursday I was dreaming of literally skipping into the office that morning, with a confirmed pregnancy and a big secret very few people would know about until our 12 week scan! The dream wasn't of me crying, in the boardroom, yet again, bereft of a baby and not a clue if I would ever have that skipping feeling. We stayed in the boardroom for what seemed like forever as I tried to stem the tears and protect the make up I'd piled on that morning.

Nobody else mentioned it in the office, but I looked like shite and knew everyone knew I'd been crying. Every time I looked in the mirror I seemed to have aged a little bit more. As I tried to rectify the make up on my smeared cheeks and to reapply mascara to my smudged, stinging eyes, I could see a face I almost didn't recognise. I'd lost a sparkle along the way. My face was bloated, blotchy and my skin seemed dull and lined. You know it's bad when no amount of make up can make any improvement and the process of applying it doesn't do anything to lift your spirits. I looked like a painted doll, a pained painted doll.

All day I was on the brink of tears, constantly holding it back. During every conversation I was distracted by my agony and in every meeting it was difficult to stop my mind from wandering and mulling over how different the meeting might have been if I'd have had a different result. It was like a big elephant sat in the room with us, that only I could see, that was only distracting me. I so didn't want that elephant to be in my life.

The week before I had arranged to meet my friend Lucy for lunch the following Tuesday and driving to work that morning, another friend, Claire, Lucy's sister, called and suggested meeting up. I was so tempted to cancel the lunch and not bother meeting up with either of them because I knew I'd just cry. I knew they would want to support me, to be there for me, but I also knew I hadn't yet reached that stage where I could be comforted and that I was still in the painful place where tears would flow freely. I didn't cancel however, thinking that pushing people away would only make the pain worse, so all three of us met in the bistro just across the road from my office.

I have always been an emotional person and all my friends and family know that I am, but I would say, that most of the time, I'm in control of those emotions and whilst I may not plan or want to cry, I very rarely let myself go. This was one of those rare occasions where not only did I cry, but I sobbed uncontrollably, in public, in front of friends. They saw the pain, the raw anger, and the desperation. I couldn't hide the hurt, the disbelief, or the frustration. I didn't want them to see me like that, I didn't want them to feel the obvious sadness at seeing their friend in so much pain but I was simply unable to control my emotions. Sat in the middle of the bistro, during a busy lunchtime service, I wiped my face with endless tissues and sobbed as we talked.

The pain that day was immeasurable as the reality of talking with friends who had been on the journey with me, really hit me. I was talking about not being pregnant, about it not working for a second time and it was real, it was now and it hurt like hell.

During the next few days I felt constantly sick with a deep aching in my stomach and an ache in my heart. I was so inconsolably sad. Nothing was lifting my spirits or lightening my mood. Everything was an effort and I couldn't shift my despair in any situation. Over and over I would be asking myself why didn't it work? Was it to do with the difficulty going in?, Was it something I had or hadn't done?, Was it because they were frozen? I had to accept that I would probably never find out but that infuriated me even more as there had to be a reason and I desperately wanted to know what to pin my disappointment on. "It just didn't work" was so hard to accept and this certainly didn't help my mood.

So now I had had IVF twice and had no baby. I was a true statistic. Two failed cycles. It had failed twice. No matter which way you said it, it always meant the same. I had undergone this fabulous treatment and I still had no second baby. My great white knight had been and gone, in fact he'd been twice and left me with nothing. My worst fear had been realised. My final card, last roll of the dice, my last hope had failed. IVF wasn't my one true solution that I had saved up for and waited for so long for. I had rolled that dice but my number hadn't come up. I could hardly believe what had happened.

My mind continued to torture me in the following weeks. All the things I had planned in my head as to how the year would pan out would now no longer be. Had I been pregnant, I would have been due in November and therefore pregnant at my brother's wedding in September. Time and again in my head I had seen his wedding photos with a huge bridesmaid and I could hear my family's voices all fussing over me and the impending new additions. Now that wouldn't be the case.

I had previously resigned myself to the fact that I was going to miss a girls' week away in Portugal for three of my friends' fortieth birthdays in September but I'd cheered myself up by reminding myself that if the reason was because

I was pregnant, then it was totally worth it. Now, I had confirmed to the girls that I would actually be able to go and had booked my flights, but I was really struggling to feel happy about the trip.

I felt my heart was breaking. It was so much more of an acute pain compared to last time and as the weeks went on it showed no sign of lifting. Last time I was so poorly that I was almost surprised to be pregnant, yet this time, this was the pregnancy that never was, that I'd lived with for two weeks, but in fact was never there. It hurt, it really, really physically hurt.

One evening after work, I walked to the car park with Dom who talked about a couple he was friendly with, who had tried IVF but had given up after two attempts and were now enjoying life, just the two of them on their own. As we got to our cars he stopped and looked directly at me saying: "You know, you might have to get used to the idea that it might not ever happen." I was shocked at his words. I was nowhere near ready to hear that or to accept that it would be the case. I told him so. I'd not finished, I wasn't ready to talk like that and didn't want to have conversations like that. I know why he said it, that he was caring and that he was just trying to help me but I thought about his words all the way home, they were ringing in my head over and over. "It might never happen?" What? Hearing those words from someone about my situation felt crazy. That was the sort of thing I mulled over in my head, in private, in the world that I hoped would never happen but to hear them out loud, said by someone else was utterly terrifying. I knew I wasn't ready to throw the towel in for sure at that moment. It was hard, it was a punishing treatment but I was sure at that moment that I was definitely not ready to accept that it was over and that it might never happen.

A few days later, I started with horrid congestion, which gradually got worse and worse and ended up as another chest infection that lasted for four weeks. People kept asking me how I was feeling and all I could muster to say was just sad, just totally sad. I couldn't shake off the sad, run down feeling, and as the chest infection took hold, my ability to crack on and give my head a shake as I was so often used to doing, simply left me.

I felt like I wanted to run. I strangely just felt like I wanted to wave my arms and legs about and somehow shake this horrid feeling from my body. I felt trapped, stuck in this sad state with no clear path to lead me to brighter days. My body felt heavy, as if I was dragging myself everywhere. It was all I could do to hold my head up some days and I felt a terrible dragging from my shoulders down my back and both arms. It was like someone had added some sort of thickening agent to my blood that made it flow slower and feel heavier as I tried to move. Everything was an effort; I felt slow and lethargic and started to hate myself for feeling that way.

I had last felt something like that when I had been suffering from depression some years before. I knew I wasn't sinking that low again, but I was starting to worry that I couldn't shake off the heavy sad weight. I knew I had no enthusiasm for anything because right now at this time, I was supposed to have been doing whatever it was you do or don't do, whilst you're pregnant, but obviously that now wasn't the case for me. So nothing was exciting me, because nothing was as it was supposed to have been.

I needed to find myself again

Jason had been going on about me doing exercise for ages but I'd always found better things to do and never found the time. I decided that I needed to break the cycle and do something to stop the rot so I called Duncan, a personal trainer we had known for years and booked a session for the following Monday.

I knew I hadn't been training for ages and on Sunday night I dragged my old kit from the back of the cupboard. It was embarrassing, a real sight and I calculated that it was probably 4 years since I'd been training with Duncan, in fact that last time was just two weeks before Zac was born.

Monday came and I had a stinking headache and had had a terribly stressful day at work. I sat outside in the car looking at my gym bag. Going to see Duncan was the last thing I wanted to do or should have been doing in my state but I told myself that having actually gone to the trouble of making an appointment, if I didn't go that evening I wouldn't end up going for weeks.

I felt really shy when I arrived at the gym. It didn't help that I walked in coughing my guts up so everyone turned round to look. My head was pounding and I looked and felt like crap.

Duncan was lovely, welcoming me back and calming my nerves. I was so pleased to have made it and pleased I hadn't bailed out. We sat in his office and talked through where I was at and what I wanted to achieve.

I needed to start to get in shape, lose some pounds but most of all, improve my overall wellbeing so that my body was fit and well enough to be ready to receive the next embryo. I knew that creating the embryo was only part of the story and that ensuring my body was in the very best condition to receive it, was one area I could focus on, control and hopefully influence. I needed that feel good factor once more, needed to feel good about myself, to feel positive and diet and exercise was certainly one way to start. In fact I started to feel excited about the prospect.

As the story came out to Duncan, the tears started to flow but pleasingly, they hurt a little less as this felt like I was starting to move forward and do something that would make me feel healthier and a little more positive. I'd known Duncan for years and so felt comfortable in his office so I wasn't worried about crying to him. I was fretting however as Jason had continued working out with him once a week for the last five years and obviously hadn't talked to him about the trouble we were having conceiving or about the two failed attempts we'd recently experienced. I respected Jason and his need for privacy enormously and felt terrible at talking so openly to someone that Jason spent so much time with. I begged Duncan not to discuss my chat unless Jason brought it up in conversation. If Jason wanted to confide in him, which he may well have done, then it should be in his own time and when he felt the need. I was desperate not to interfere with that for him. Duncan promised and I believed him and it felt good to know what we discussed in his office would stay in his office. We then did half an hour of exercise with what was left of the session and it immediately felt great to be back in the old routine.

When I got home I felt energised already and really felt like I'd turned a corner. I told Jason all about my session with enthusiasm, that was until he looked in disgust and disbelief at what I was wearing and saw my work clothes folded in the carrier bag I'd used as a gym bag. I felt embarrassed at the look on his face, knowing exactly what he was looking at. He was adamant that he was going to get me some brand new kit and a new kit bag to take it in. I think he was more than a little intrigued by my attire and my carrier bag but it showed how little I cared about such things at that time, because I really hadn't been that bothered!

As soon as I got home I started to look at my food differently. Just being with Duncan and spending time in his gym had inspired me to get my act together and ditch all the high sugars and treats that I had started to rely on and tell myself I needed. They were the last things I needed as the lows that follow a sugary high were coming all too frequently now and weren't doing anything for my overall mood.

The morning after I felt fine but on Wednesday I was aching all over. I couldn't shake off the need to vigorously shake my arms and legs and really release some tension. I still had the feeling of needing to run, to scream and shout and was desperate to get fully into my exercising and free some physical demons. During my lunch hour I went across to the shopping centre to hunt down some new gym gear. Not sure how long I was really going to commit to exercising, I didn't buy much and didn't spend too much but as I walked out of the store feeling more than a little giddy at my purchase I bumped into my dear friend Julie. It was a real rarity to bump into her in town and we were both really excited so decided to go for a coffee and catch up.

I told her all about how I'd been feeling, about visiting Duncan and showed her the bits of kit I'd just bought. Julie had been a professional dancer all her adult life and after having her children, she became a dance teacher and more recently a Zumba teacher. She told me all about her class, which I confessed had always sounded a bit beyond me in the past, but right there and then over our latte and muffins, I found myself promising to go to her Wednesday night class! I was excited but scared at the same time! What on earth was I getting myself into?

The class was everything I expected but so much more. Jules was like a machine up on the stage shaking her booty and showing us all the moves. She was amazing. Not only was she fabulous at doing the moves, she was exceptional at telling us what to do early enough and kept the repetition going so that we could easily learn the routines. The music was funky and happy, the moves were fun and liberating and it felt great to be moving all over the hall letting myself go. It was the most I'd moved in months and it felt fantastic. I was smiling all through the class and even found making mistakes hilarious. It was utterly exhausting but the most fun I'd had in ages.

The next day, I couldn't move but I felt great and knew I couldn't give it up.

The following week, I went to the gym and Zumba again but by now the congestion had really settled on my chest and though I hacked through both sessions, I loved it all the more.

It was a huge effort to get away from work on time to make it to the classes but the bigger wrench was having an evening away from Zac. I rarely spent time away from him, especially as I was working full time. After collecting him from nursery at 6.15, we would have almost two hours together every evening and I cherished every minute trying to be with him as much as he and his growing independent streak would let me. Even having one night off from him was a huge wrench but now with two nights I really felt like I was punishing him and cheating myself. Of course, he and Jason enjoyed terrific 'dad and lad' time and I always got back to be able to read to him and tuck him into bed so he probably didn't even notice, but knowing I was taking time out away from him, to hopefully prepare myself for another child, felt really selfish and cruel when I so wanted to enjoy the gorgeous child I already had.

As I started to feel better about myself, I did start to feel however, that the small sacrifices twice a week could possibly be worth it. I had more energy, felt generally brighter and I thoroughly enjoyed both sessions so I felt invigorated when I got home. I was looking better too, starting to tone up which in turn also made me feel better.

Plus, by this time, Zac had a new distraction, his two baby sisters! For sometime Zac had entertained us with his imaginary friend Roger, and now it seemed, out of nowhere, he also had baby Tilly and baby Jessica. They would come to play and Zac would have to go out of the room to change them or feed them. Sometimes they would just cry and cry and other times he'd tell us the funny things the babies had done and we had to laugh too, which wasn't hard! They would come home from nursery with him and sit next to him in the car. A few times I had to ensure they had their belts on too! He would talk to me about how nice their names where and asked if I liked those names. But by far the funniest moment with 'the babies' was when he came in early one morning upset because baby Tilly had been sick all over the cot and Jason had to go in and pretend to clean up and tidy the make-believe cot before he calmed down! Jason duly did so, whilst I stayed in our room crying with silent laughter. Jason was such a fabulous Daddy, why the hell couldn't we share his love with more children?

We couldn't help but wonder however, whereabouts in Zac's mind the two babies had come from in the first place, and whether he had heard anything that we had been talking about that had stimulated those thoughts. Whilst it was cute and amusing to listen to his stories about them, I also found it really troubling that he should be having to rely on made up baby sisters to entertain him. He was so loving and gentle towards his imaginary babies, he showed he'd be a gorgeous big brother, which made his play all the more painful to me as I'd listen and admire his caring ways.

Baby Jessica and baby Tilly were a big part of our lives for quite a few weeks and whilst some of the things Zac came out with were hilarious and kept us amused, the very presence of those two baby girls was a stark reminder of what I felt was missing in our home. I knew I had more love to give other children, but I felt Zac was also showing us that he too had so much love and laughter that could be shared with a brother or sister. Jessica and Tilly seemed to leave after a while, though were occasionally mentioned and whilst having to do the extra work to accommodate the babies had sometimes proved frustrating, when they did finally disappear, I'd find myself missing them and asking how they were!

Work during this time weighed heavy. I could hardly muster any enthusiasm, I couldn't concentrate and I really didn't want to be there. The actual work, clients or colleagues weren't the problem, we were doing great and the company was going from strength to strength but I found I wasn't leading with my heart and therefore everything seemed forced and a struggle, which was a way of working I wasn't really used to.

Emma was on holiday, and one lunchtime I noticed one of the young interns walk sheepishly back into the office, looking as if she'd been crying. I'd taken her under my wing as I really felt she could do well for herself if she worked hard and she was a really lovely, polite girl. She knew all about my treatment and she had offered really kind words, wishing me well and saying what a great mummy she thought I already was. I called her into my office and sat her down asking if she was all right. She was protesting that she couldn't tell me, but after much persuading she finally broke down and told me something I certainly wasn't expecting or was prepared for. She had just done a test in the shopping centre toilets and found out she was pregnant.

The pregnancy was neither planned nor prepared for and, having found her feet with her internship and with her immediate career path mapped out with more certainty, it was certainly not what she had in mind at this time in her young life. As someone grieving an inability to conceive, it was certainly not what I felt I could cope with at that time either. That said however, I was grateful that after the initial feeling of a blow to the stomach, I was able to muster a huge strength to take her in my arms and soothe her. The poor girl was beside herself, she was in shock and she was terrified about the immediate future in telling her boyfriend and family. She had also been terrified at the thought of telling me, given she knew how much I had been trying for a baby and I really felt for her as she sobbed in my office and apologised over and over for having to tell me in this way. Thankfully, I was able to calm her, to support her and advise her on what to say and what to do later that day. I suggested she go home straight away and try to let the news sink in, as she was in no state to stay in the office. I really felt for her. Just as she thought she had landed on a great work opportunity that would set her up with her career and make best use of her skills and studies, she was thrown off track. She was such a sweet girl and I felt so, so sorry for her.

That said, with no Emma to share the responsibility of looking after her, I wasn't feeling too great myself. After she left I took myself outside onto the street to take some deep breaths of air and try to regain my composure that had been so strong and was now threatening to crumble, as I tried to make sense of the injustice I felt was being served.

First I had to support someone through an abortion, now another through an unwanted pregnancy. Two unplanned babies that were conceived without thought or want, whilst I was undergoing expensive, painful procedures, to try to do exactly what they did without thinking. Playing the scenario over and over in my mind was now causing me to gasp and shake as I started to react to my immense jealousy and anger at our differing situations. The intern thought she wanted her baby, which was a small comfort but still, it felt that God was playing games with me and they were terribly cruel games that deeply hurt.

As he was a business partner, I had agreed with the intern that I should tell Dom, especially as I was sending her home. As I told him later that day, I could feel myself breathing fast and gasping my words. "I can't cope if she stays here, she will have to go after her internship, we can't keep her on if she's pregnant, I just couldn't cope with seeing her growing belly!" It was horrid to say but it was how I felt. Dom was shocked at my words and told me not to be silly but I really felt that afternoon that watching her pregnancy progress, with her baby growing inside of her, would be too much to cope with. That was just too much and I knew immediately that it was a situation I needed to ensure I avoided. It was hard to admit how I felt, but it was so overpowering and it was how I was genuinely feeling. I could not cope watching her belly grow bigger.

My worst fears were avoided however when sadly, just a few weeks later she miscarried. Strangely, all I felt was utter sorrow for the lost baby and the new hurriedly planned future the intern was now not going to have. I never wished harm on her or the baby and having accepted that, one way or another, I was going to avoid being around her; I was really saddened by her news. She was just a girl, who having had the shock and upset in finding out she was pregnant, now had to cope with the shock and upset of a miscarriage and I found myself wrapping my arms around her once more, this time completely feeling her pain and trying my very best to continue that support. It was eventually pleasing however that she bounced back surprisingly quickly and from there went from strength to strength with her career and I'm pleased that to this day, we still have a silent connection from those weeks when we shared so much.

Over the next few months we had a stressful period at work with lots of change, which I never like. Three employees left, we had three major clients who all suddenly had wobbles and as Emma, Dom and I knuckled down to re-steady the ship, I struggled to stay strong as I felt I had to concentrate on being able to concentrate! Having stability at work had enabled me to turn up each day, put a hard day's graft in and come home to look after the family, whilst still having the brain capacity to plan our extended family. Now, with the additional work and strain of a busy period at the office, there was little time for anything else and I felt like my life started lose focus and lose direction. My period seemed to be taking ages which added to my stress levels and there was too much work on that was far too stressful, to allow me to even think about starting the treatment again. Yet I knew that was the one thing I was counting on to get me on back on track. For the first time, I actually started to hate work and all that it was taking from me. I had always had a feeling that my career had cost me my ability to conceive in the first place, and now it was taking away the time and head space to be able to get myself in a position to try for another baby.

I missed the clinic, the contact, the drugs, the focus, the feeling that I was just a few steps away from having another baby, even doing the injections. I missed it all and longed to be back on a programme. I missed the plan and the formality of taking one day at a time, counting down to harvest and transfer. Being on the programme felt like a definite step towards having a baby, rather than the airy fairy wasteland of diet and exercise that I currently felt I was stuck in and getting nowhere fast.

A friend gave me a little voile bag of gemstones that were each meant to symbolise various elements of good health and fertility. Both her sister and sister-in-law had also been recently trying to conceive and she had bought all three of us a little bag each. I was really touched by her thought and gesture but as she then told me both of them were now pregnant and followed that up with " So now, there's only you!" I felt a growing rush of frustration. As if this little bag was all it was going to take to make me pregnant too. It wasn't a great time to be given this gift or to hear that comment and I was confused by my obvious delight that she should care enough to think of me and the fury at the money making, thoughtless idiot that created such a bag who had no thought at all at the hurt their superstitions might cause. A bag of bloody coloured stones indeed! I did keep the bag however. Of course I was too suspicious and nervous that they just might work that I dare not throw them away! If I ignored all the other emotions the bag of stone stirred up, it was a lovely thought and her good intentions were much appreciated. It was nice to think someone was rooting for us.

Jason and I decided that we should try to cheer ourselves up by investing in the house and redecorate some of the rooms. We hadn't spent a lot of time or money since the house had been first built some five years earlier and some parts were looking decidedly tired. This brought us to the point where we decided the time had finally come to move Zac out of the nursery and give him is own 'big boys' room. He would move across the landing into what was a spare room, which meant that we needed to build cupboard space and tidy the room we used as an office and general store room to make that a second spare room.

Overall we ended up decorating three rooms, having the paintwork in the nursery freshened up and then having the full house repainted. The project gave me a focus and gave the family a feel good factor, as we got excited about how nice the house was going to look with all the changes.

An interior designer gave me some ideas and a mood board for the downstairs and I ordered new wallpaper and curtains for the lounge and dining area. We had floor to ceiling cupboards built in the new guest room, created a office area and bought new bedroom furniture and accessories for Zac.

After looking at pirate themed rooms for months and deciding on various elements that I thought looked really cool and perfect for Zac, he informed me that he wanted a football room and certainly not pirates. There was no persuading him, so football it was. I refused however to have green curtains, walls or bedding and was adamant it wasn't going to be Hull City's black and amber, instead I found a gorgeous mix of wallpaper, bedding and curtains in various blues and reds with the highlight being a huge navy silhouette of a footballer on one wall. I had his first Hull City shirt framed, which was signed by Dean Windass, along with our programme from the Wembley final where Deano scored, which we put on one wall too. He absolutely loved it and he especially loved his two huge drawers under his bed, one for fancy dress and one for football kits. It was all designed around him, for him, and he loved everything about it.

Then it hit me. We were moving Zac out of the nursery. We had an empty nursery, a situation I had been trying to avoid. What was worse was that the painters had taken down all his nursery paintings from the back of the two doors in the kitchen before I had had time to take them down myself and when I came home from work that night to see two freshly painted, white doors, it was like someone was stripping the house of my baby. Removing every trace from the house. I broke my heart that night and I can honestly say that the act of someone removing those paintings still hurts me to this day. I wasn't ready. I hadn't realised they would need taking down and I hadn't prepared myself for all that was going on. It was a huge milestone in his growing up and our family dynamic was moving forward and further away from babies.

That weekend we spent Sunday afternoon putting Zac's new furniture together with all three of us involved. It was lovely spending time doing something together and as it was all starting to take shape Zac was getting more and more excited, to the point where he was starting to get hyper and get on our nerves!

We had three funky box shelves for one of the walls and I put 'Nan nights', his old comforter, in one of them and I proudly showed him where he could keep it. He was incensed at my suggestion and told me that it was not for his new room and that it was for babies. I pleaded with him to hang onto it in his new room and that he didn't need it in his bed but it could have a new home on his shelf. "You don't need to snuggle him darling, you can just have him up here looking after you, see?" Again he told me I had to take it back to the nursery for babies.

After what seemed like the longest pause, I walked out of his new room and across the landing back into the nursery, holding 'Nan nights' and I placed the frayed worn out teddy back on the shelf with all his other baby teddies. I felt like I was betraying 'Nan nights' that had previously spent every waking and sleeping moment with Zac, so much so he was mostly threadbare. I was desperately trying not to cry but it felt like the final act in saying goodbye to my baby. He didn't want his comforter anymore and we had nobody else who would love it. Zac's words cut threw me and I had big heavy sobs caught up in my throat. It all seemed so ridiculous but yet so painful. Jason had obviously had a word with Zac, as he followed me into the nursery and gave me a hug. My little four year old boy was comforting me about a bloody washed out, worn out teddy. It was ridiculous! And yet, as ridiculous as it seemed, it was another seemingly insignificant, innocent moment that broke my heart and reminded me of what I was missing. I missed my baby boy and both myself and 'Nan nights' were missing having a baby to love us.

That night as I lay with Zac in his new big boy bed having our usual little chat before he closed his eyes he said: "Mummy, why were you crying? Do you want me to have that teddy in my room?" I smiled at his innocent question and I had to agree with him that it was for babies and that I was crying because he was growing up and a I felt a bit sad that 'Nan nights' didn't have anyone to love it. I suggested I would pop in every now and again and say hello so he wasn't lonely. After Zac then said that he would have it in his room, I was quick to reassure him 'Nan nights' didn't belong in his big boy, football room and I tucked him in, squeezing him good night. My baby boy was so grown up in so many ways these days.

Finishing Zac's room had taken all day and I found it really hard. I felt like I was being forced to do it and as I transferred his clothes across the landing, every step seemed heavy and hard to take. Every so often Jason would give me a hug or smile at me and crack a joke to make me laugh. It just felt like the hardest time and it physically hurt. I felt like I was erasing any trace of babyness from the house, even though Zac had outgrown the nursery, the decoration and the cot bed, months before.

Later that week I got my period. Another milestone. Another cycle. Another chance.

The following weekend we finished moving all Zac's clothes and bits and pieces, which gave us the opportunity to clear out a load of old stuff from nursery. We changed the room round so it wasn't just as it had been and now empty, we put a spare sofa in one corner and left the door open so it wasn't closed away. Having the cot bed as a bed rather than the cot also helped, and in fact it made it a nice guest room for when Minnie or Zara came to stay.

This time, just one week later, with hormones realigned, it didn't feel like we were losing a baby, rather that we were preparing for a baby and getting ready for our future. Instead of being sad at throwing things away, I had starting thinking that I wouldn't put that on my new baby or that something was too old or too worn for a new baby. Just seven days later, the same chores now seemed liberating and positive and I started to feel lighter, brighter and physically more capable of picking myself up. My mood seemed to thrive on the thought that now Zac needed to move into his new room to make way for a new baby, which was a complete revelation compared to my dark mood and thoughts from the previous weekend.

Take three, third time lucky?

A ndrew and Kate had set the date and I was over the moon to have been asked by Kate to be a bridesmaid. Three years older than them both, and with Kate having a sister, a daughter and lot of young nieces, I hadn't really seriously considered that I might be a bridesmaid and was completely thrilled to have such a super special role. Kate had decided on our full length, one shoulder, blackberry dresses and I absolutely loved them.

I went to the shop to order mine and the owner was advising me to order a 12. I'm small yet I've never been skinny, but I have always been a size 10. So I was confused why the lady advised on a 12 when the sample size 10 I was trying on seemed to fit. She suggested the size 10 shop dress had been tried on many times and that a brand new one sent from America might be a little bit tight round the bust and hips? Once sent, if a 10 didn't fit, she couldn't guarantee a 12 would then arrive in time for the big day, but if we ordered the 12 they could take it in. I knew I was a size 10 and that a new size 10 would have fitted perfectly but at the back of my mind, I also knew that there could be chance that I would be three months pregnant at the wedding and therefore it was probably wiser to order the 12 just to be on the safe side. Afterall it would no doubt be my bust that would expand first if the last two attempts had been anything to go by! And so we did order the 12, much to the smug delight of the shop owner, though she didn't know the real reason I agreed with her. Making decisions based on the possibility of me being pregnant made me feel giddy. I was really excited to be ordering a bridesmaid dress but I couldn't wait to squeeze into my size 12 with a big fat belly and magnificent enlarged bust!

Having confirmed the date of my period, we had arranged a consultant appointment and attended a few days later. We had hoped that, as promised, the team would have the findings of their audit meeting and would have some advice or recommendations to offer us. As soon as you realise the treatment's not worked the first question is 'why?' Was it something I did or that the clinic did? A thousand questions run through your mind and you consider every little thing that you did on every day through the process, wondering what it was that might have affected the result. That one Bacardi you had, the day you had back-to-back meetings, too little sleep, too much stress, or too few fresh vegetables…. And so it goes on. You question the clinic's actions, did they prescribe the right dose of drugs, did they make sure the embryo was healthy, did they put it back in properly or drop it half way in? Some questions are sensible, some suspicions are ridiculous but one thing that is constant is that there is never a precise conclusion. Nobody can really tell you why, nobody knows why. There may be theories, considerations and suggestions of slight changes in your treatment if you choose to go again that may help, but really, there is no answer. It just wasn't meant to be.

That said, and knowing that we would probably never find out, did not stop our excitement and eagerness to hear what was discussed in the audit meeting by the whole team, who we were told would be discussing our case. We met a new consultant and made our way to one of the familiar meeting rooms with great anticipation.

As it was, the consultant we saw had neither been in the meeting, nor read the notes made by those who were, before our meeting. To make matters worse, once the three of us discussed our last two attempts and he flashed through the audit meeting notes, he actually disagreed with the recommendations the meeting had made and recorded!

I was furious. He was totally unprepared for our meeting and now, was throwing us into further confusion as to what to believe and how best to proceed. I could feel the heat rising in me, the tears pricking at my eyes and my voice getting higher as my throat and mouth started to dry up.

I explained that I didn't have anything against him as a person and I apologised for being curt and to the point, but that in my occupation, if I hadn't attended a previous meeting and turned up to see a client without having read the minutes, my firm would be sacked on the spot for being so ill prepared and unprofessional. It was a complete waste of everybody's time and a huge blow to our emotions.

What was the point in having the so-called 'audit' meeting if the conclusions weren't digested and passed on to whoever was over seeing the case? Why even discuss it if any decision made was going to be ignored or contradicted? Where were the lessons being learned or acted upon in our best interest? We felt totally on our own and like a number on a production line. This wasn't something we were taking lightly and it was going to cost us at least £4,000 to do another cycle so we wanted to take the very best advice possible. I could hardly believe that we were sat there feeling so lost and angry. Not only did we have no clue on the best next step we were now starting to lose confidence in the team that was supposed to be helping us. It was a truly horrible feeling.

We were both really angry and we let it be known, but the consultant promised that the team would all get their heads together and write to us with the best way forward.

The inital money was gone now, spent, we wouldn't see that again. Two cycles down and two large cheques spent. We had to get our heads round digging deeper into our savings but at this stage we were more than ready to literally put our money where our heart was, if not our mouth. We knew it was a lot of money, money we could have spent on ourselves, on Zac or kept as a safe nest egg but right there and then, there was nothing I wanted to do more than spend any money we could get our hands on, on another cycle. It felt right to take another financial gamble.

Some days later we received their letter advising us that we should try a fresh round again but reduce the levels of drugs so that we avoided hyper stimulation. There wasn't a great deal of information, no great lesson learnt but it was enough to give us the confidence to try again.

Round three was starting and by now, I was ready for it. This was it. To those few people who knew we were trying again, I was saying "Well they say, third time lucky!" and I really felt this was it. In my own head I could reassure myself with the facts that the first one had taken but we lost it because I was so poorly; the second didn't take because they were frozen and therefore this time, with what we had learned and the change in both sets of circumstances, we were bound to be successful. I could placate my nerves with reasoning as to why it hadn't worked the first two times but I couldn't dampen my excitement at my confidence that this time would work. I went to pay the invoice and collect the drugs from the clinic. I was excited to finally get hold of the big brown, non-descript paper bag full of drugs!

The injections started again, the bruises appeared again but none of it dampened my spirits this time.

Later that week we went to look round Zac's new primary school, which felt really surreal to both of us. We were introduced to his new class teacher who I immediately fell in love with as she reminded me of my first reception teacher, Mrs Sales, and I instantly felt she would love and nurture my little boy. Zac had such a strong, loving relationship with the girls at nursery I was fearful that the formality of the school setting might be a shock to him and one he might shy away from, but I was completely put at ease by the Headmaster and Mrs Wordsworth. Whilst I was quite excited for Zac and knew how ready he was for this next step, it was again another reminder of how leaving nursery was another step away from my baby and the thought weighed heavy on my mind all week. It was all happening at the same time and it was really, really troubling me.

Work started to improve as clients settled back down and we had two new girls start as Account Managers. They were really nice girls, with excellent upbeat attitudes, which was something we had missed in recent months. There was a new buoyant atmosphere amongst the team brought on by the new recruits and you could feel the positive impact it was having on everybody. I was working with both girls on different accounts and as I knew I would need their support at work when my treatment started I decided to immediately tell them my circumstances so they had as much preparation time as possible. We didn't really discuss it after our initial chat but I felt better that I was being honest with them. I hoped they felt more confident having been immediately forewarned that they would be holding fort for a week in a few weeks time. It felt like a new era, a new chapter and it was already feeling good.

My diet was fantastic and I was eating a whole range of healthy and super foods that were making both Jason and I feel a lot better about our overall well being. I was still going to see Duncan at the gym and Julie at Zumba each week. I was starting to show real muscle definition in my arms and legs, a well-defined core and my clothes were looking and feeling much better on me, which in turn had a positive impact on my mood. I began to feel more confident than I had in ages. My overall positivity made me feel that the time really was right for another baby and that our stars were all aligning. Work was settling down, team holidays were working out well for me to have time off, the stimulation injections were going well, I'd carried on acupuncture and acupressure twice a week, I was feeling fit and healthy and I didn't have a chest infection or cold this time either. I really felt there was nothing else I could do to be anymore positive or practical at that time and that feeling in itself was really empowering.

The girls were still planning on going away to Portugal for one of our friend's 30th birthdays and there were about 20 of them going for 4 days of fun and mayhem. I was really gutted not to be going but then I felt almost weirdly positive that it would be worth it and I shouldn't be sad as there would be plenty more trips in the future. Of course I did feel a pang of sadness that I should miss out, especially as they came back with hilarious stories about what they'd been up to and a nice glow from the sun. I just needed to focus on the here and now and my life was a world away from theirs right now.

My girlfriends and I arranged a night out in Leeds where we drank cocktails, played silly games and danced somewhat irresponsibly in the restaurant, but we were having a great time together and nobody bothered us. I'd set my alarm on my phone to remind me to do my injection. I couldn't miss one and for half an hour before kept checking my phone for the time to ensure I didn't miss it. Discreetly I made my way to the ladies and thankfully avoided anyone joining me to reapply lipstick or sort their hair out.

Stood in the cubicle in Harvey Nichols toilets, I filled the needle and stuck it into my tummy. It hurt like hell that night, most probably because I was tense, but I'd managed to do it without fuss and returned to the table. Nobody knew, nobody needed to know and I carried on enjoying myself happy in the knowledge that again I was another injection down and another step closer to my ultimate happiness.

I was halfway through a session with Duncan when he said he would be off for the next 2 weeks and we worked out that this was therefore my last session with him before the transfer, even though that was nearly a full month off. I was so shocked! I had been training and working out knowing that the treatment dates were getting closer but to feel that they were almost here was a massive shock and suddenly I didn't feel ready. I wanted to shout, "Don't finish yet, I'm not ready, I need more weeks to prepare, I can't stop now, I've got more work to do!" I could feel my eyes pricking. I tried to get a grip of how irrational those thoughts were but tears poured down my cheeks and neck, as I gritted my teeth and continued countless crunches across the ball. The time would soon be upon us.

I had started the stimulation injections the week before I was off and I was now having scans regularly. The more I went to see the clinic the closer I felt to the team and the closer we were getting to the all-important transfer. Being back on a programme made me feel in control, on the journey and that was as calming as it was nerve wracking.

After complications last time I was scheduled for another mock transfer and dilation where they had decided they would stretch my cervix to help enable the catheter to pass through without potential problems. That morning I tried on four outfits before deciding what to wear as I just wanted to look smart and presentable. Jason said I was dressing as if I was going on a night out and I remembered previous times and that each time I got nearer to my treatment, I always tried to dress smartly. It felt like it might be how you would dress if you were receiving a certificate or medal I would imagine. It made me smile at how ludicrous but typically 'girly' this was!

Our appointment was 8.00am. I was really apprehensive this time as I got lost in thought about the previous complications and I sat behind my curtain with Jason, preparing for the worst. We waited for more than 2 hours, which was particularly anxious for Jason who hadn't officially taken time off work and had thought we'd be in and out. His anxiety made me anxious and after some time I started to get cross. He was on his phone constantly keeping plates spinning and when he wasn't he sat agitated, fidgeting and tutting. I whispered loudly that if he was that bothered he should have taken the full morning off as I'd suggested and that I wasn't going to let him make me any more nervous so he needed to either lighten up or leave. Of course I was nervous too and I was already worked up but neither of us could do anything about the delay, we just had to wait.

We recognised the very deep baritone voice of the consultant we were seeing that day, and we could hear his dulcet tones booming across the clinic area. At least we knew he was in the building, though he didn't sound like he was preparing for theatre. Finally, after what seemed an eternity, we were called into theatre where the nurses were also quietly getting angry about the senior consultant being so late. The whole scene was charged and not very comfortable at all, despite the nurses trying to relax us both.

As I sat on the bed, whilst we waited even longer for him to actually arrive in theatre, we were talking to Debbie the nurse, who was always warm and good-humoured. We were talking about Prof and how funny he was and we were all reminiscing about his hilarious antics at the last transfer. She told us a few of the stories he tells patients to calm them and his favourite one, that she had heard a thousand times, about the woman dressing up in stockings and suspenders for her transfer because she wanted to get 'into the moment'. At least I didn't go that far! We were all laughing loudly as the senior consultant finally walked in.

After all the worries from the previous transfer, this time they were straight in, so much so I left like a fraud, with all the clinicians waiting to do a cervix stretch now all stood down. I couldn't believe it. Thankfully two of the nurses confirmed to the team that they had been in the previous procedure otherwise I would have thought I was going mad. Yet it was clear this time I didn't need dilation or numbing and now we all just hoped that my cervix would stay that way until transfer for real just one week later!

Attempt number 3! This was it!

It was the Queen's Jubilee so it was a double Bank Holiday and I was worried that the clinic wouldn't scan me regularly enough across the weekend to avoid hyper stimulation. I started to panic that the royal celebrations would throw a curveball in my cycle. However I was assured that the clinic was open for scans so once again I began to feel positive and confident. On the Wednesday, I had the first scan and as the drugs this time were starting on a lower dose, I was really worried that I wouldn't be stimulating at all. I climbed onto the bed next to the sonographer almost too nervous to lie down for fear of hearing that I hadn't responded at all to the low dose. I lay back, took deep breaths and gritted my teeth.

The scan showed I had responded and was stimulating well. So yet again with another hurdle jumped, Jason and I were feeling really optimistic and more importantly, I was feeling really well.

By Friday I had started to have a bigger tummy once more and this time really sensitive nipples. The whole of the front of my body was really painful and any contact made me reel back in agony. Poor little Zac would get pulled away from my arms as he leant in for a cuddle or wriggled on my knee. I didn't want to push him away, I particularly didn't want him to feel that I'd pushed him away, but the pain was overwhelming at times and it was an automatic reaction. I learnt new ways to hold him, carry him and have him snuggle next to me that didn't press on my tummy and avoided my tender breasts.

The scan showed I already had as many follicles as the first fresh time (27) and they were already just as big at this early stage as they were at the end of the first. This time however, I also had a little bit of fluid round my ovaries which was causing some concern and meant they would have to keep a closer eye on me.

That night I worked till 9pm in the office determined to get as much finished and leave detailed notes for the team, so that I could switch off as if I had gone on foreign holiday and was uncontactable. I had booked the next two weeks off work to spend time with the family and properly relax ahead of the transfer. I felt it was vital this time to try to really switch off from everything else. I wanted to enjoy time with Zac and Jason and not complicate my thoughts or emotions with anything to do with work. I had always taken my job seriously and taken any issues to heart, so unless I completely switched off, I knew the smallest query would trouble me. The transfer became my absolute single focus. We had so much invested in this third cycle and not least our life savings but nothing was more important.

I had worked so hard over the previous weeks to complete a thorough handover to my colleagues and was relieved to be happy with the status of all the projects, but as soon as I walked out of the door, I immediately lost interest in work and appeased myself that I could pick up any issues, should they arise, when I got back. For now, I was on leave, I was happy with the work I had put into the handover and the team were more than capable of looking after the clients.

That weekend we went to my aunt's 60th birthday and 25th wedding anniversary party, which was a really lovely occasion and it was great to see the family. The party was in their local church hall and was perfect for the younger kids who could run around freely. Zac loved running around with his cousins Zoe and Elin and he looked really cute in a smart pale blue shirt and shorts. He had photographs hugging my Mum and I could see she was bursting with pride and love for him. That day in particular, I couldn't wait to have more children. We all had so much more love to give and Zac was a shining example of how much love your child could give back.

By this time however, I was literally struggling to walk as my enlarged ovaries once again felt like huge boulders in my tummy. I had to literally waddle around the hall or simply sit down and take the weight off my feet as the weight of my engorged follicles and the increased fluid weighed heavy in my stomach. Once again I really felt pregnant. It was quite a nice feeling in a strange way and although it was very painful, it was weirdly nice to think that soon I might be waddling with a pregnancy. I'm sure it was only that thought that stopped me crying with pain that day.

I tried to keep an eye on Zac, Minnie, Zoe and Elin as they played in the two large rooms but it was almost impossible and I had to rely on Jason to watch them as I sat to one side. Mum had told my Auntie Pauline and cousin Paula that I was having treatment and both had quiet words with me and gave me a squeeze. I was tearful both times as I felt so emotional about it all and was obviously in so much discomfort. Yet it was also strangely easy to smile whilst describing the treatment and where we were up to as I really felt it was a small price to pay for the baby we were about to have. It was like I was saying yes, it's painful and yes I'm having difficulty moving today and if I didn't love you so much there is no way I would have come out today, but, it is all part of me making a baby and I am thrilled at the prospect. Of course I didn't say all of this to them but the thoughts made me inwardly content despite my discomfort.

By that Sunday evening however, we were all back at my Mum's house and I could hardly walk and was very breathless. Andrew and Kate were also staying and as we all sat round in the lounge, I didn't feel I could enter into the conversation. I could hardly breathe let alone talk. Zac and Minnie were playing lovely together and I was dying to spend time with them but I couldn't find the energy or the strength to get off the sofa. I kept saying to Jason that I was fine and that I could cope but it was when he finally said maybe I shouldn't have to feel I was 'coping' with anything that we rang the IVF emergency helpline and explained the situation. We were told to stop stimulating that night and to come in the following morning for a scan, even though it was Bank Holiday Monday.

That evening as I cuddled Zac on Mum's sofa, I had to keep telling him to be careful of my tummy. "Mummy you have a huge belly, it's got a baby in it!" he said laughing his head off. I told him: "It hasn't got a baby in it darling" to which he replied: "Well it looks like it has, it's massive!" Charming but observant! He thought his words to me were hilarious. Once again, a part of me really wanted to share our secret and tell him how hard I was trying to have a baby for us all. It upset me that I couldn't have him on my knee at the moment and for the last few weeks hadn't been able to carry him down the stairs first thing each morning for his breakfast, as he still so loved me to do. It seemed that I was all too frequently telling him to get off me or saying no I couldn't cuddle, hold or carry him. Very soon he wouldn't want me to carry him or he would be too big to carry anyway and it tore at my heart that I was wasting this precious time when I could be holding him. It hurt knowing I would never get that time back. I hoped he wouldn't pick up on the constant negative comments I always seemed to be making to him at the moment, be it protecting my tummy or making him walk by himself. I so loved that close contact and prayed that once all this was over and I had the baby, that he would still be small enough and needy enough, that I should be able to hold him in my arms once more. I never wanted that feeling to ever end and hoped I wasn't wasting the last few weeks when it was possible. I stayed with him that night long after he had dozed off in bed, whilst I sat in great discomfort, just listening to his snuffly snores and stroking his back in the way that he loved.

The next morning we set off for the clinic and we had to take Zac with us. As it was short notice we didn't have anyone to look after him. The irony of being stuck for childcare when we were going to the fertility clinic didn't escape us. We thought long and hard about what to do but decided it would be OK, as you don't really see anyone when you attend for scans and the waiting room is generally empty. It was typical that this was the first and only time the waiting room was totally packed with couples! We had explained to him that we were all going to the hospital as I had a big, sore tummy but that I was ok. We told him that this was where he had been born and taken from Mummy's tummy, a fact which he found so interesting, it distracted him from the fact that we were there in the first place. All the way there in the car we had to answer endless questions about how and when he was born!

As we all sat in the crowded waiting room I was really proud of him quietly playing with his dinosaurs and pirates and I had a huge urge to stand up and say to everyone, "look what can happen, look at our miracle boy, you must have hope!" Yet on the flip side, I also felt really guilty for bringing him in and though he had been a really good boy we quickly decided that Jason should take him outside. Jason said later that he too felt really awful and awkward and although one girl sat on her own kept smiling at us, we couldn't help but wonder what they would all be thinking and hoped we hadn't upset anyone with our ill-thought through action in taking our child along with us.

I waited for ages to be called through and then had the longest scan I had ever had, as I had so many follicles. By now there was more than 30 and they were all pretty large. The kindly Sonographer described me as a "sonographer's nightmare" and said she hoped they didn't have any more like me in the waiting room! It was typical that the only time there were so many delays and only time there was a queue was when we had Zac with us.

Jason popped back in but I was still waiting to see a nurse to hear their thoughts once they had analysed my scan. I thought he'd be frazzled but he was quite calm and apparently Zac had been a good boy. He had explained to Zac that Mummy still had a sore tummy and was now going to see a doctor, which he took well and didn't seem unduly worried about. Worrying about Zac was the last thing I needed today but it wasn't an emotion I could just switch off. Even though I knew he was with his Daddy and seemingly unfazed by the trip to the hospital, I just wanted to get back to him quickly and reassure him that I was fine.

After being called back in, it was explained that my follicles were large and that my ovaries were the size of Jaffas but that the fluid seemed to have disappeared and this was a good sign. They took more blood and I would have to await results. I laughed with the nurse as my arm spat blood everywhere as she removed the needle and then wouldn't stop bleeding. I've never been good with blood! You would think I would have been used to needles by now, but it seems I wasn't and the sight of so much blood was definitely a different matter all together. I took deep breaths as I held a swab on my arm to try to make it stop, as I certainly didn't want to go outside to Zac with blood pouring out of my arm. I needed to sit for a little longer too whilst I tried to cool down as the effect of seeing so much blood had made me feel more than a little faint.

I was told we would be scheduled for retrieval that Wednesday or Friday. I was hoping it was Wednesday as the weight in my tummy was unbearable. I wanted it to come as quickly as possible and wanted as long as possible off work following the transfer so Wednesday was definitely my preferred day. I slowly waddled out, still holding my arm and went to find my boys. Once again, I heard myself telling Zac to be careful, this time of my arm as well as my tummy, as he excitedly tried to hug me and show me where he had been exploring. He was unscathed from his visit to the hospital and I just hoped those waiting in the waiting room were too.

Later that Bank Holiday Monday, which was Jubilee day, we had friends coming round and we planned to go to the street party in our village. I felt huge and I struggled with the usually easy 15-minute walk to the village green. As we walked I told my friend I'd been for a scan that morning and she squealed and squeezed me with a strange delight. I realised she was several steps ahead of us and thought that I was pregnant! As I let her down gently and told her not yet, I desperately wanted to finish the sentence with "but we're on our way."

There weren't many places to sit on the village green but I had to keep stopping and sitting on the floor to get the weight off my legs. As the party went on around us and we all stood in a crowd for a commemorative village photo, my phone rang and the name of the clinic flashed up. The blood test results showed that my Estradiol levels were very high, hence my current discomfort and therefore we would have to coast for a few days and wait until Friday for retrieval. I was instantly disappointed but the news was not unexpected. Denise wanted to consider the file properly but she too was at a family Jubilee party so sent me a text to say she would call me to discuss the plan in more depth the following morning at 10am.

I went back to Jason and our friends where Zac's friend Harry was proudly informing everybody that Zac had changed his name to Steven (as in Gerrard) as his Mummy was having a baby and he wanted it to be called Zac! We all laughed as they both confirmed this to be the case! How thoughtful our little boy was and how comical the pair were together. We had already seen that he had made the girls at nursery change his name on his peg to Steven but we had only assumed this was after his footballing idol and had been unaware as to his ulterior motive! I updated Jason on the news and he like me sighed knowing that we had really expected that outcome all along.

We wanted to make the most of Jason having the week off so planned a few days out and went to Sundown Adventure Park the following day. It was a visitor attraction designed especially for children under 10. It seemed to take forever to get out of the house and knowing I was expecting a call at 10am I was probably more than a little tense. The call came at 10am when it just so happened that we pulled into a fuel station where you are not supposed to use your mobile. Perfect timing! Despite my ungainly enlarged figure I clambered up the grassed embankment to get a clear signal and so that I could hear Denise properly. I will never forget that phone call, it was so important and yet there I was, breathless from climbing the steep bank, with the phone to one ear and my hand to the other ear as the breezy wind whipped my hair all round my head and blew a gale down the phone!

Denise confirmed that the levels hadn't come down but they hadn't gone up either so she considered that to be a positive and could therefore confirm retrieval for Friday. We were thrilled at the prospect and relaxed for the rest of the day. The park was huge and I literally waddled the length and breadth of it. Anyone looking at me would have assumed, as indeed I felt, that I was 6 months pregnant. I had an enormous belly, enormous round boobs and I was waddling as if I was with child. Again it was a nice feeling imagining what it would be like to be really pregnant and as uncomfortable and painful as it was right now, it was also a lovely feeling that I enjoyed all day.

Zac loved the miniature village and whilst he had a great time going on all the rides with Jason, I did feel a twinge of sadness and regret that I couldn't join in a much as I would have done normally for him. I had to sit out most of the time and it felt like he was getting used to me not getting involved and it wasn't something I wanted him to remember his childhood for. I was and wanted to still be an active, fun Mummy and it troubled me that day that it had felt like I had been moving away from him more and more during the last few months.

The place was naturally full of young children, babies and it seemed like another pregnant belly would greet me around every corner. There were bumps everywhere and I so wanted to be part of that gang. It's always the same when something is new or on your mind, you then see it everywhere for days later and on that day I swear that pregnant women were purposefully placing themselves in my path. It was an enjoyable but difficult day and one where I really felt like I'd taken one for the Davies team in managing to get through it. And yet, I felt strangely optimistic that our journey was all but over and we were within touching distance of our positive ending.

On Wednesday we had planned to spend the afternoon at The Deep aquarium and in the morning I needed to go to the hospital for another blood test, then I was scheduled to have acupuncture and we would all have lunch together. The blood test was completed quickly so Jason and Zac were able to stay in the car but whilst I was in there, I had a call from work asking if I could pop into the office as one of the girls was off with chicken pox and we had a radio deal that needed checking and signing. Going into the office wasn't actually stressful and I didn't enquire about any other clients or projects but it did mean I had to cancel my acupuncture session, which I was furious about. It felt like the story of my life. Plans always mess up when there is the slightest opportunity to do something for me! It was typical but we did manage to grab lunch in the bistro across the marina from my office and then headed to The Deep.

To take in all the exhibits you naturally need to walk through the attraction and once again I found myself waddling in pain and sitting out whilst Jason spent time with Zac touching starfish and seeing the fish up close. I felt horrendous on that day and was completely exhausted but I really wanted the boys to have a good time. I wanted Jason to enjoy his time off and feel he had spent it wisely and wanted Zac to enjoy his adventures doing something different than playing football. I was desperate to go home though and was so relieved when we got to the end of the tour and were finally heading back.

By Thursday I was tired and felt really quite low. I was starting to worry as my tummy was really sore and by now I was struggling to muster energy or enthusiasm for any day trips no matter how much I wanted to for the boys' sake. I had got to the point where I couldn't pretend or muster a second wind, I was really struggling and it showed.

As it was a nice day, Jason suggested we go to a local golf club for a coffee and see his friend who was the golf pro there. When we arrived however, Zac was fast asleep in his car seat and I didn't want to wake him, as I knew he needed the rest so we didn't stop and carried on to Yorkshire Outlet Shopping Centre. There we enjoyed a nice lunch and had a little wander round the shops and as it turned out had some really lovely family time together. We bought Zac some nice tops in Ralph Lauren that were smaller versions of some of Jason's which he was thrilled with, but that was where his good mood unfortunately ended! Every shop we went in after that he wanted to buy Minnie something, which was really cute, but clearly not feasible. It did show me his caring, loving nature again though and I couldn't wait for him to be thinking of his own sibling in the same way. It showed what a lovely big brother he would make, that was until we told him we weren't going to buy something today for Minnie. His good humour and pleasant nature was now forgotten, as the combustive mix of being told no, being sick of shopping and starting to get tired, turned him into a little monster. We cut the afternoon short and made our way home, with both Jason and I asking each other what on earth we wanted another child for!

Third time lucky

The next morning, Friday, I awoke feeling good in myself though still really sore and swollen. Zac has woken in a good mood and got dressed with little fuss or refusal, which I was pleased about. His opinions on his wardrobe were getting increasingly strong but not particularly in good taste and there were days when I'd send him in a real mash up of clothes but I'd agree to anything as long as it would get him out of the door. Gone where the days when he hadn't a clue what he was wearing and I could dress him as I wanted.

Those clothes were now all boxed up with labels on detailing 3-6 months, 6-9 months and so on. When I'd first started putting the clothes he'd outgrown away, I'd carefully place them in the boxes feeling slightly giddy thinking about the next little one that might soon be wearing them. As months and eventually years wore on, every time his drawers started to burst or you could see too much of his socks under his too-short trousers, I reluctantly cleared out his wardrobe and felt queasy in the knowledge that the items may never see the light of day again. Not least in our house anyway.

That morning though he was too busy nattering on at us about football and trying to count down the days to the football training. He got dressed quickly, ate double the usual breakfast and gave me a lovely big cheery hug as Jason took him off to nursery whilst I got ready. What huge joy that boy brought to me every morning.

When Jason returned, we then made our way to the clinic. It was a strange journey for me that day because I was bursting with excitement at the prospect of moving forward with the retrieval at last but I was also extremely uncomfortable and in a lot of pain, which slightly dampened my spirits. I waddled into the Women's and Children's Hospital entrance towards the

IVF clinic on the ground floor. It's the exact same entrance used by those going upstairs to the delivery suite and for the first time, I felt a real rush of excitement about everything that happened in that hospital. I couldn't wait to come through those doors again and head towards the second floor!

It felt good to laugh as Caroline welcomed us in and noticed that I was wearing flat shoes, which I very rarely did. She then recalled how out of it I had been after my first retrieval and we all laughed as she reminded us how Jason was almost carrying me out in my sedated state! That was exactly why I was wearing flat shoes this time!

As ever we received a friendly reception from everyone in the clinic. Once again it felt exciting and I couldn't wait to get started. Painful as it was, it was still a very important day and I was giddy as we made our way towards to my bed in the waiting area. We asked if we could move beds to the one we had been in on the first retrieval. We weren't really superstitious but the first cycle had worked and we would try anything to make this cycle work. Jason squeezed my hand as I made myself comfortable on the same bed.

Whilst I was having a canula needle placed in a vein in the back of my hand, Jason went off to perform and do his bit! Once again it struck me how utterly unfair this process was for women!

This time we quickly went into theatre and the procedure began. Perhaps there was more sedation used because this time, I couldn't remember anything about the retrieval. Jason told me all about it as I sat on the bed in recovery with my much appreciated cup of tea and chocolate biscuits. This time they had been able to successfully retrieve 14 eggs and they were all good quality. Though I was obviously awake and alert, I can remember nothing about leaving the hospital or getting home!

That weekend, I could hardly move so great was the pain in my stomach. I literally couldn't switch from one bottom cheek to the other on the sofa. I spent the next three days lying there almost motionless. If anyone else sat close to me and caused the sofa stuffing to move even slightly, it sent sharp shooting pains through my stomach and caused me to shout out in pain. My belly was enormous and literally looked like I had a football down my dressing gown. I kept trying to get up and walk to try to relieve the pain but the bearing down in my nether regions and the swaying and stretching of my muscles across my stomach were too unbearable. I had to revert to sitting with my legs up, daring not to flinch to try to get some relief. Despite my stomach ulcer history and being advised not to take Ibuprofen, I actually took two that

Sunday as I couldn't bear the pain and thought any stomach pain I would get from the tablets, wouldn't be any worse than the pain I was already in. A pint of milk later to line my stomach and I'd had the first Ibuprofen that I'd had in more than 10 years.

I also had a terribly tickly nose and non-stop sniffles that I was desperately hoping it was just the effects of the oxygen and not the start of another cold. I could not be ill again, I just couldn't bear to have to fight off another infection whilst going through the next few weeks; I really needed to stay well. I was frantically Googling looking up the effects of oxygen and whilst the tickliness didn't seem to be letting up, I was somewhat relieved to learn that the nasal tubes in my nose and oxygen were indeed probably the cause. It seemed there was always something to worry about!

I was also constipated by now and had loads of wind, which also gave me stabbing pains. I managed to get to the toilet and have the smallest poo but it was like having a baby and the pain right through my body was excruciating. I was crying in agony and by now as it approached Sunday evening, I was starting to worry that if I remained in such a bad state, that they might not want to, or be able to put the embryos back in. I couldn't understand it; I'd had half the dose of drugs but had more and bigger follicles this time? I was obviously hyper sensitive and I just hoped that this wouldn't affect my state of health and ability to receive or keep hold of the embryos.

I called the clinic first thing on Monday morning and was thankfully told that we had 10 good quality fertilised embryos and I felt ecstatic. Ten was a super result at this stage and I was excited that we could probably have a couple put back and then perhaps be able to freeze some. It was tremendous news and once again I was flung back into an optimistic mood at what I felt was another positive sign on what I was hoping was a successful journey. The pain suddenly seemed worth it, if not welcome, and I felt more able to deal with the discomfort and the emotion of denying Zac any hugs much better for the rest of the day.

Wednesday came round so slowly but when the morning finally arrived I rose with some trepidation. There was one final hurdle to cross before transfer and I just hoped my embryos had survived the last two days and were still strong. Annabel, a lovely embryologist called early and told us that from ten, we now just had one embryo that had reached blastocyst stage and was strong enough to transfer. There would be no freezing this time. There was just one survivor. Just one left. Just one chance. I was totally shocked. I was terribly upset for the other nine and couldn't understand what had happened to them in the last two days!

Considering they do such a technical, scientific job, the embryologists were always surprisingly brilliant and empathetic when they called you to discuss how your embryos were doing, particularly as it was not always a positive call to make. I spent 20 minutes talking to Annabel asking countless questions, trying to understand what had happened to my ten chances. I can't remember any questions and I can't remember any of the answers but something she said that morning struck me and has remained with me ever since. In fact they are words that I repeat often to any friends who are also trying for a baby. "It's a harsh reminder of just how much of a miracle getting pregnant really is." She was right. It's easy to watch Jeremy Kyle and think you just need a Bacardi Breezer and wham, bam you're up the duff. Yet despite so many girls appearing to get pregnant apparently so easily, the stars still need to be aligned and it is still truly a miracle to create new life. The Bacardi Breezer Brigade are either lucky or unlucky, but it doesn't take away from the miracle that still happened to create that child, whatever the situation or circumstances. Annabel was right. Getting pregnant was nothing short of a miracle and I needed to remember having this treatment was no guarantee. Through my tears down the phone, her words reassured me and grounded me. She reminded me that I only needed one embryo after all to have a baby. She was happy that we had one strong one that she was confident in transferring later that morning. I just needed one and I had one. It had been a shock but that had passed and I needed to give my head a shake, get dressed and go and receive my one, healthy, strong, embryo.

Jo texted me and I updated her on the one single embryo. I told her our angels were with me and she texted a photo of Zara dressed as a fairy and said her little fairy would be with me too. It made me smile and made my tummy turn. Again, it was a stark reminder of how precious life is and what a miracle birth is, so, with my fairy photo saved onto my phone as a screen saver, I left the house once more feeling really positive.

On the 20-minute drive I was really nervous as I was still in a great deal of pain and discomfort and desperately didn't want Denise to say I was too sore for transfer. I once again tried my best to walk straight and tall and to keep everyone distracted from my discomfort with the usual nervous, cheery chatter.

Given the severity of the OHSS symptoms again during this cycle, the team suggested only putting the one blastocyst embryo back in. There were others that weren't as good quality that could have been transferred but the team felt that with one exceptionally strong one that clearly stood out from the rest, putting more than one in would be too risky for my health, particularly if then, more than one embryo should transfer successfully and turn into a multiple pregnancy.

I absolutely hated always having this conversation in the theatre whilst in my gown, sat on the bed. I felt vulnerable, emotional and whilst the team were caring and giving their very best advice, I really felt cornered and put in a position where I had to agree with what they said. I really wanted to have two put in if that meant I had the slightest chance of being able to get pregnant with just one baby, but with so many authoritative, qualified people around me all advising to stick with one, once again, through floods of tears, I conceded and agreed to just put the one strong one back in. It may sound daft that I should consider putting any poorer quality ones back in, but I just wanted the greatest chance and if it took putting 8 back in for just one baby to be created then that's what I wanted them to do, even with the risk of becoming terribly poorly or becoming the UK's first Octomum! I just wanted the very best chance.

As it was, once again I bowed to their experience and somewhat to the pressure of the situation I was put under. I couldn't understand why you didn't have the conversation over the phone in the morning in the comfort of your own home, or even in the waiting area behind your curtain before you go into theatre. The time and place of that conversation left me feeling extremely helpless and it felt like I was handing my destiny over to someone else to decide and dictate. During parts of the conversation I felt utterly helpless and forced down a path I didn't really want to take. This naturally made me angry. I already felt powerless at my situation and now having these people take more control and further decisions away from me, just added to the sheer frustration and desperation.

There was a huge push in the infertility world to reduce the number of multiple births. In my very few saner moments I understood that having one healthy baby would indeed fulfil all my hopes and dreams and that there are so many more complications with twins or indeed larger multiple pregnancies. Yet I can honestly say that 99.9% of the time, having the conversation with me at that time, warning me about multiple pregnancies, was absolutely futile. In my head, I wanted to increase my family. With the emotional, physical and financial strain of repeated rounds of IVF, I wasn't sure how long we could go on and I knew that even if we were going to be successful this time, that this would be then be our last time and we wouldn't go through the treatment again in the future for a further child. One baby would be great, two would be fabulous and even three would be a complete blessing and give us the longed for noisy, busy house full of our children.

The nurses' warnings about financial strain were wasted on me, as I knew we'd cope, cut back and somehow survive through our love of our family. We were already under huge financial strain just to undergo the fertility treatment given the lack of funding. It was hugely stressful to be handing over thousands and thousands of pounds to have our family when in my opinion so much NHS funding is wasted. It had really started to get under my skin that just because we had a child, meant that we weren't eligible for any funding for fertility. It wasn't like we had 'spent our allocation' on our first child as we had paid private for that too. Our issue was unexplained so it wasn't like it was 'our fault' either. It was wholly unfair and whilst we could find the money, it was beginning to be a huge wrench and source of worry for us.

Their caution about the health risks to myself and any multiple babies and myself were also received with little interest though, as I believed they were over exaggerating and above all, I just thought they were being targeted by the health service to reduce multiple births and they were only interested in their single birth percentage rate. I was convinced that it was all driven by the politics and the Government trying to save money in the NHS by having one less person too look after in future life. As a hard working, tax paying citizen, this only sought to fuel my determination to have the very best chance of a large family that I could have, no matter whether the pregnancy resulting in one, two or even more babies. It was my family, my body, my decision and I was livid that new, external forces were trying to take control when Mother Nature was already doing her damn best to prevent me from having more children.

I was having to pay in full for this bloody treatment, why didn't I seemingly have a say in how it was spent? It was a minefield of a debate but sat there I felt so angry that despite even paying for my treatment myself, I couldn't decide how many to put back.

Perhaps the IVF team found that having the conversation in this manner, in theatre, just as they were about to transfer, ensured the more successful outcome to make certain fewer embryos were eventually put back. This would then result in the desired outcome of fewer multiple pregnancies, but it was something I hated about the process and that feeling of being hijacked and controlled in this way would stay with me for quite a few days thereafter.

That said, when Annabel put the photograph of our blastocyst embryo up on the monitor in the corner of the theatre, a huge wave of positivity and love washed through me as I stared at my baby for the very first time. Just a tiny pin prick of cells and yet my whole future was up there on the screen. "Wow, hi there little one" I whispered as Jason squeezed my hand and wiped the lonely tear that was slowly rolling down my cheek. I couldn't wait to feel that my little one was inside me so I could love it and care for it and hopefully feel it grow. I listened to the team once more about safely retaining a pregnancy with one healthy embryo and fell in love with my little emby instantly. I knew they had our best interests at heart really.

As emotional as the experience still was, I felt really strong and positive this time. I felt physically ready, mentally strong and we had learnt so much from the last two times I felt sure we were going to make it this time.

I was hugely relieved that they finally did do the transfer. The scan beforehand showed that my ovaries were extremely swollen and there was still quite a lot of free fluid but Denise decided it was safe to go ahead and I was so thrilled that finally, our one little embryo was safely transferred.

The two week wait that wasn't

We returned home where I rested and pottered round the house, trying to take it easy. I allowed myself to dream a little and revisited my little list of names that I'd been compiling and editing for nearly 2 years now. I added a couple on, crossed a few out and rearranged the order of preference. It felt great and I felt more than a little giddy at the reality of what I was doing. Not only did the name have to go with Davies but it also had to sound nice with Zac. Zac and…. Just trying to come up with a little brother name and little sister name was exciting for me.

Of course when I asked Zac he said he wanted a little brother called Steven, which in my view was actually a huge relief because he'd have been quickly shot down if he'd suggested Gerrard. Girls names he was a little more relaxed about but suggested Jessica, Tilly, Millie or Mummy. All very cute but not exactly what I was thinking. Hhmmm Zac and Steven….it wasn't sitting right either really!

The pain and discomfort in my tummy started to ease off and I could move more easily as the days went by. It made it easier to hug Zac and snuggle next to him in his duvet when I put him to bed. I longed for him to remember hugs and cuddles with Mummy and not being asked to avoid my chest or tummy or to get down from my lap. In so many ways he still felt so much like my babe in arms, I never wanted to lose that feeling no matter what happened in the future and I certainly wanted him to remember himself in my loving arms. Those damn drugs! My damn sore body!

On the Saturday after transfer, one of my aunties had arranged a get together for all the family on my Dad's side, which included all my aunts, uncles, cousins and their children. We are extremely close though we don't see each other often and I was determined not to miss it. As we hadn't had a family wedding in ages, there had been no occasion to see everyone so I really wanted to go. I did make it, though I felt quite tender and uncomfortable still.

Everyone was there except one of my younger cousins, who by total coincidence was also having IVF and was having her transfer that very day! I was initially really surprised to learn that Debbie too was having treatment but knew instantly not to ask too many questions to my Aunt and Uncle as they were obviously concerned and didn't want to talk about it. I understood and asked them to give her my love and told her sister that if she wanted to talk to me or ask me anything that she should call me at any time.

I had the strangest mix of emotions on hearing the news about her treatment. I knew she would conceive. I knew in my heart of hearts that she would be successful and I was excited for her knowing how much she had always wanted to be a Mum and this would be her first. Yet I was also tormented by the thoughts that this was our third attempt and questioned would it really be fair if she was successful after just one attempt and we were to be unsuccessful yet again?

The huge weight of guilt at having these thoughts dragged me down. I hated these thoughts, I was turning into a monster! I knew that whatever happened to Debbie would have no bearing on my life, my cycle, my potential pregnancy. The overwhelming guilt at questioning the fairness of someone else's pregnancy was nothing to the guilt of desperately wanting mine to work out, knowing that someone else was still waiting to know the joy at having just one child. I loved Zac, my family loved Zac and Debbie loved Zac as her second cousin. Here I was greedily wanting another baby when Debbie had yet to conceive a first. I felt greedy, I felt guilty but most of all I felt ashamed at all these bitter thoughts going round my head. It was horrid, like poison and it was starting to drive me insane.

Of course I didn't want Debbie to experience the pain of the treatment not working, and whilst I'm not proud of the fact, I knew that afternoon that I would find it really, really hard to deal with, if she conceived and I didn't. Surely with our dates just days apart and with us girls being so close, that would be a really cruel outcome? Surely too cruel? I had to believe that we too would therefore be successful. Another reason to think that this time we would have our baby.

I had extra long and extra hard squeezes from a couple of aunties who knew what had been going on which was lovely and welcome, though I had to move away quickly and change the subject, before their sincerity and kindness moved me to tears! As it was June, and my brother was getting married the following September, as we left that evening we all signed off with 'See you at Andrew's wedding!' and I smiled to myself as I thought 'yes you will and I'll have a lovely bump when you do!'

The next day was Monday morning and I was back to work. I had carefully planned and cleared the early part of the week's diary, as I still wanted to ensure I relaxed into it and took it easy. It wasn't to be though, as Emma said she had a viral migraine and therefore couldn't do a presentation that was scheduled for later that afternoon and that I would have to do it. It was a client and subject I was familiar with but it was in front of 60 people and on my first day back! Whilst I could do it, it wasn't the sort of tummy churning, nerves-inducing activity I was hoping for on my first day back, just three days after transfer! It wasn't exactly following a textbook post-transfer plan.

To make matters worse it was at a venue owned by a guy I had fallen out with some years before and had not seen since, who as it turned out was also there doing a presentation. Again, not the most relaxing of circumstances for me. I read through the notes, did some editing and as it turned out delivered a great presentation, though it was certainly not the best-planned or most relaxing first day back at the office! It had been unavoidable but certainly not ideal. I left and went home early as the venue was closer to my house than work and tried to rest before collecting Zac from nursery at 6pm. It was going to be a takeaway dinner night!

The following morning I had a 'show', followed by slight bloody streaks in the mucus.

I called the clinic and spoke to Caroline who confirmed my worst fear. She did say that given the timing, just five days after transfer, that it could be just a late implantation bleed and that I had to relax and try not to worry. I was terrified but tried deep breathing for the rest of the day and tried to distract myself by throwing myself into briefing meetings updating me on client projects.

On Wednesday morning I awoke to loads of blood. It was most definitely a period now. There was no doubt. I texted work to say I wouldn't be in with little explanation other than I had a period. I was in total shock.

I knew instantly. It was a numbness, a sinking cold feeling that needed no explanation or clarification. I was bleeding. Anything that had been there couldn't possibly still be there.

Not even a week on from transfer and I'd lost it. Had I lost it? Had I ever had it? I called the clinic and this time couldn't control my tears as I cried to the familiar, caring voice that I was fully bleeding and was in no doubt that my period had arrived. The nurses said once more that they were really sorry, but that I would still need to do the pregnancy test the following week to make sure.

I didn't go into work that day. I cried practically all day.

Looking back I think it would be a really interesting study to watch me on my own that day and plot the different, changing emotions as I tried to come to terms with what had happened. Shock, grief, anger, despair, back to shock at the severity of the anger I felt and that the situation was real and so on. Time and again I would hear myself screaming through gritted teeth as I dropped to my knees and cried into the carpet, then with fists clenched thrust myself up and howl into the air as if the answer or cause of such pain was above me and I wanted them to know how much I was hurting. Surely this is primeval, animal instinct but it is certainly one of only a handful of occasions when I have literally let rip and let my emotions out in such a way. And yet this time, the screaming, howling, clenching of fists and grinding of teeth was relatively short lived as most of the time I simply walked round the house like a silent zombie, sobbing at times but mostly letting the silent tears fall as I stared out towards the garden or buried my head under pillows.

The grief and anger are certainly triggered by the realisation that the dream is over, but it's easy to forget about the huge impact the drugs and hormones are having on the body when the period arrives, so on top of feeling horrendous mentally and emotionally, I was also feeling horrendous physically. In the past, I have had experience of receiving terrible news and grief when someone close to me has suddenly died. Yet in this situation you have a huge physical reaction to hearing terrible news, but your body is also already under super intense pressure, so it is perhaps no wonder I was often surprised at how draining those first few days in the aftermath really were.

On Thursday morning I texted work again and arranged to take another day holiday. My head was banging and I couldn't see how I could possibly be of any use to anyone, let alone dress myself and drive to the office. The realisation that it was all over took only moments to hit me the moment I woke up that morning and I pulled the duvet round me trying to get comfort or perhaps protect me from any more hurt. I couldn't get through the day feeling this way. I didn't have the strength to worry or wonder what people would think if I just stayed hiding away in my bedroom for the next week, I just didn't know how to move forward and function when I felt so utterly bereft and broken. It was as if my emotions ran through my veins and right now those veins were snapped, ripped, unable to flow freely and enable me to get up, walk, think, let alone speak or smile. Getting through a normal day seemed a million miles away from where I was and how I felt as I lay there and I really didn't care how ridiculous that may have sounded. I couldn't find it within me to start to even think about how best to rebuild my broken spirit. My headache was immense, my whole body seemed heavy and the despair I felt deprived me of any energy to lift my head and try to deal with the situation.

I was dozing on and off for a short time and just lying under the bed covers, lost in thoughts feeling utterly desolate, when after some time my thoughts began to clear and I started to grasp at some level of real world clarity. I started to ask myself, what else am I going to do all day? How much more time could I take off work when I was running out of holidays? Was I just going to cry all day? There was work to be done, a house to keep and of course, Zac to look after. My sanity was starting to return, even if my energy and willpower were a little slower to show themselves.

By lunchtime I had managed to shower, change, slap my make up on and, though still feeling like a wet kitten, I managed to drive to the office. I sat in the car for at least 5 minutes trying to muster whatever it was that was going to get me out of the driver's seat and up the steps into the office and survive. I took deep breath and got out. As I got to the path, one of the designers, Andy, was coming out to go to lunch. He stopped, took me in his arms and said "Oh Helen, I'm so sorry, are you alright?" I pulled away and sniffed "Andy don't!" and put my head down to walk towards the door. Andy is much younger than me and though I knew he really had no understanding of the detail of what we had been through, knowing he was just so sorry that I was upset was enough to make me tearful at his lovely consideration. He knew I wanted a baby desperately and I knew he knew how much I loved my Zac. His hug and words meant a lot but I thought were the last things I needed. As it was, it was perhaps a good job he did that outside as I then walked into the office, feeling like I had broken the seal and got over it. I was then able to say: "Don't ask me if I'm alright because Andy already has and I'm not" and we were all able to laugh.

That day, I threw myself back in work with full force and nobody asked again if I was all right. I had cried for a whole day the day before and now, all that heartache had to be closed into a box and I had a life to get on with. I had business partners, clients, employees, husband, son, friends and family who all needed me right now. What's more, they needed me sane and fully functioning.

Reality bites and hurts

It happened surprisingly quickly. I was becoming hardened. I began dealing with the situation remarkably quickly. Previously it had taken me weeks to recover, if not months. I had felt so utterly bereft and deeply sad that I found it impossible to function.

This time was different. I was devastated of course but I was more in shock and angry than sad. The hope that I had held onto for what seemed like so long, was just all too often batted away and crushed. What was the point in being positive? I felt silly at having felt so optimistic and believed in all that Positive Mental Attitude bullshit! I could not have been more positive this time or prepared any better and it still hadn't helped.

What struck me this time was the feeling of total, utter helplessness. The horrid reality that no amount of money, effort or positivity could help me. I had nothing more to give, there was simply nothing more I could have done and still, I couldn't conceive. That feeling of helplessness was horrendous and scary and the world suddenly seemed like a huge, challenging place that I felt threatened by. I wasn't in control of my destiny and despite every fibre in me doing everything it possibly could, I still could not control the outcome.

Never in my life had I ever felt like that. For years after my Dad left, we had very little and the feeling that debt and doing without gave me was one of being extremely scared and vulnerable. It was a gut wrenching fear that scarred me but also shaped me and made me wholly conscious that if I was ever going to have anything or achieve anything, then I was on my own and I would have to fight for it. And fight I did. Professionally and personally I worked my ass off and had some terrific jobs, started great businesses and made terrific friendships. As a competitive runner, in my school years, I knew I had to forget everyone else, run my own race and give it my all for those few seconds when it counted. If I prepared and trained hard and if I focussed on the day, I could win it, and win I often did.

I've always felt I could have choices and achieve what I want if I just put my mind to it. If I work hard, go for it and don't stop till I get there. I can't afford to buy a Range Rover, but it's never stopped me from believing it's within my reach and ability to do so. I don't live in a million pound house but that doesn't stop me from getting up each morning believing it is within my potential to do so one day. I don't have the figure or face that I would ideally like, but I do believe that if I could be arsed to spend the time on myself and really wanted to put that bar of chocolate down, that it is within the realms of possibility that I could look like someone I would want to look like. I had always had an inner grit that never took no for an answer, never accepted I couldn't do something and an in-built belief that anyone could achieve their desires if they just put their mind to it. My primary school motto was 'only your best is good enough' and I had grown up thinking that if I worked hard and gave my best I could achieve anything. I had always believed it and it had stood me in good stead. And then all that changed in one day. Now, that foundation was cracking. I had given everything and I had nothing left to give. Yet I had achieved nothing.

The realisation that no amount of money that we'd spent, food I'd eaten, alcohol I'd not had, caffeine I'd avoided, vitamins I'd taken, exercise I'd worked hard on, acupuncture, acupressure, reflexology, reiki, positive thinking, relaxation and rest, not to mention the drugs and medical intervention, could make me pregnant, rocked my very core. It wasn't just the feeling of having given it my all and it still not being enough, it was the shock that it seemed no amount of money or effort would ever give me the result I wanted and the realisation that this could be it forever.

We had paid £15,000 on all the treatments so far but would it have changed the result if we had paid £150,000? I had spent every day of the last 8 weeks focussing entirely on my diet, exercise and rest, but would it have had any different outcome if I had done that for 80 weeks? I couldn't fight any harder. I couldn't do anymore. I had more money but that wouldn't help. I was utterly shocked and grief stricken by the fact that it really was just fate, and it was no longer a case of how hard I fought for it, it was now completely beyond my control. I longed for that control back. I craved the feeling again that I could perhaps affect the outcome in some way and I felt immensely terrified at the realisation that getting that control was never going to happen.

Trying to make sense of it all

I struggled to control the shock and the fear and I didn't feel I could speak to or see anyone. The shock had blown me off my feet and I needed to try to make sense of the new way I had to view the world and my place in it, before I tried to digest superlatives from those around me trying to console me. It wasn't just that it hadn't worked now; it was much bigger than that. It was now a real possibility that it might never work and if it did, it would purely be down to luck and therefore the question was whether we had the finances or the strength to go through this any more when luck was all we had to rely on. Like someone saying spend ten thousand pounds and you can win a million if your ball lands in the back of the net. But you can't kick it, someone else has to do that for you. No control. Could you afford the money or the stress to take that chance? I'd have said yes instantly a year ago but after three kicks I doubted that we could risk any more. The prize was great but the stakes were high and now getting higher. Taking away any effort that we could put in made the dream seem less of a reality and the risk far greater.

With three failures and especially with the last one, in my eyes, without any agreeable reason, I really felt like a statistic. One of those women in Women's Own with a crazy life story that you read about but never really believe exists, only now I was starting to and was beginning to think I'd be next to grace their pages! We'd failed three times. Three times. Not third time lucky at all. No reason, no explanation, it had just not worked.

From the moment we put our first foot on the IVF journey, I had never thought for a moment that this was where we would end up. I can honestly say, even if I may have talked about it at times, the thought that it might not work, did not really figure in my plans or seriously cross my mind. And now there I was, one week later, doing a bloody pregnancy test just to finally prove that I was definitely not pregnant. It was just a formality, but needed to be done, but I felt angry almost at the stupidity at wasting a test. And yet, numbness quickly took over. Sorrow was quickly overshadowed by a deep, black sensation that blanketed any feelings I may have normally shown.

I called the clinic calmly and updated them. Once again I heard how really sorry they were and I knew they really meant it and felt so sorry for us but this time, I didn't cry, didn't feel any real emotion as the numbness just about enabled me to function. I agreed to make an appointment to go in and meet with Prof after my next period. Perhaps the only feeling of sorrow my mind allowed me to feel at that time was actually for their team and the clinic's statistics. At that time they were the leading IVF clinic in Europe in terms of success rate and I felt dreadful that I should be one of those to dent that success rate when they were such a terrific bunch of people who showed utter devotion and dedication to help people like us. Other than that, I felt and showed nothing. My emotional tank was empty.

I didn't want to talk about it with anyone. We'd tried our best, it didn't work, end of. What else was there to say? I'd find myself repeatedly just saying, "it's just shit" to try to end a conversation or relieve a friend who was struggling to find any words of consolation. There weren't any and if there were, I wasn't prepared to listen right now. I had much bigger concerns that I was battling with at that time. Like how the hell was I going to get through the rest of my life when I now believed my fate was sealed in all areas and nothing I ever did would be able to affect or improve it. Life is just down to luck. It was a terrifying thought.

At that time, the enormity of the shock and grief was perhaps almost too much to deal with and so my whole being just shut down that emotional side of my body and spirit and numbed any feelings at all. I didn't cry but now I also didn't laugh. I didn't get too depressed but I also didn't get excited about very much either. And yet, on a positive note, I was getting up each morning, I was functioning at work and I was getting through each day, hour by hour, which was a bloody blessing given how dreadful I felt.

It was almost like I couldn't even begin to start to deal with the grief for fear of how huge, overwhelming and consuming it would be. If I opened the floodgates there would be far too much to deal with. This third round failing was just the final straw that broke the camel's back. Just talking about this round would open a wound so huge, so old, so raw about all the years I had desperately wanted another baby, that I was afraid it would finish me off and leave me in a straight jacket.

Not being able to make a baby was a big enough issue for me, but now, also dealing with a scale of helplessness I had never experienced before meant that trying to deal with the upset and seek help was definitely out of the question. I couldn't afford to take the time out of my life to deal with it and to try straighten out my head and my heart. I had a business to run and a little boy who needed me, not to mention a husband who was hurting too and who needed my arms round him as much as I needed and welcomed his around me. No, this time, the numbness had to remain to keep me going, to get my family, my business and me through each day to the next.

Life without a bump

Zac became the focus of my life and a positive element that brightened my days. Here I was with pain in my heart from the children I didn't have, but with a beautiful boy in my arms early each morning and at the end of each day. In those days and weeks, I more than anyone knew how lucky I was.

It was hard to talk to anyone openly and honestly about the pain I was feeling by now. Those around me would always try to cheer me or make me feel more positive by referring to Zac, how gorgeous he was, kind, great at football, cute and so the list when on of all Zac's great attributes that I was apparently blind to. I knew I had a fabulous kid! I knew I was lucky! I just wanted to scream sometimes that I wasn't daft, I knew he was great, that's why I want more! It was futile. Too few people understood.

They'd question why I was putting myself through all the heartache when I already had a child. They'd tell me I'd be crazy to give it another go and say surely I wasn't thinking about another attempt. They'd suggest it was unfair on Zac to spend all our money when we could spend it on his future. Friends, family, even random acquaintances who knew little of my circumstances, were all so concerned but couldn't see past the fact that I already had a child. Nobody questions whether a desire for another is reasonable when you try to conceive naturally. You may need small intervention but Mother Nature's calling is just as strong, in fact I'd argue stronger when you're in the fight.

As ever my beloved boy was football mad and I really enjoyed watching Euro 2012 with him as he followed his favourite players and their countries through the competition. He baffled Jason and I with his knowledge and facts about goals, players and results. He was just four years old but with the football trivia of a Match of the Day pundit! He had also recently started to get interested in American Football on the TV and made Jason and I roll about laughing one morning when he walked into the bedroom wearing just his bright blue cycle helmet saying he was going to nursery as an American Footballer. He did indeed go to nursery with his cycle helmet on and whilst I persuaded him to also put shorts and a T-shirt on, he did insist on putting his shin pads over his shoulders for added effect. He looked utterly ridiculous but completely hilarious! In his eyes, that morning, he was going to the Superbowl and I loved him for it.

Zac was about to go through a hugely important transition in his life as he graduated from nursery and prepared for big school. In so many ways, nursery had prepared him wonderfully and he was ready for school, and yet in others, he was still so tiny and seemed too young to be leaving. He had been there from five months old, five days a week and was very much an important part of their family as well as the fixtures and fittings!

His last few weeks were utterly divine as the staff indulged his character; made a fuss and made each day so memorable for him I'm surprised he didn't chain himself to the gate. His utter love of football was embraced by the team who held a special football tournament on the back field. Zac was one of the captains, picking his team, leading them out on the field and they even had a pretend stretcher such was their dedication to indulge his passion for the sport and his imagination. Zac's team won after he scored 13 goals and they ended the afternoon with a cup and him being paraded round the field on the shoulders of the staff. They even had water, or pretend champagne, to squirt in his face. I was amazed and loved the attention to detail but loved it more when they told me that he had been helping them plan it for weeks. He really was a joy to be around and I felt huge pride that afternoon, as I knew how much my lovely little boy had touched their lives and how much they were going to miss him. We had been very, very lucky to find such a wonderful nursery as The Old School House and I was going to miss them greatly. Over the years, I had watched Zac's friends' parents come through the baby room with their baby brother or sister in their arms, to pick them up from the main room, as I walked through the main door on my own for Zac. How I longed to need to go to the baby room again. How I had hoped, dreamed and believed that our relationship with The Old School House would go on long after Zac left. It was clear Zac was getting ready to fly the nest and leave nursery but to the contrary, I was pretty sure that I wasn't ready. I didn't want it to end. I wanted to carry on coming, but in a matter of weeks, I would have no reason to come and the thought of that chapter ending made me extremely sad.

It was around this time that I went with Zac for his first half day at school. The combination of my sadness at leaving nursery and anxiety at what I felt was like handing my child over to the State, made me feel really nervous and jittery and I tried my hardest not to let Zac see this. I talked about how exciting it was to meet new friends, learn new things and he seemed pretty relaxed as we parked up and walked towards the gate. As we got closer however, his grip on my hand got tighter and he pulled himself in towards my body a lot closer. I really didn't want him to be afraid and I slowed, stopped to hug and reassure him, then we carried on with our walk into the playground.

As we met Mrs Wordsworth and had a look round the classroom, Zac instantly relaxed and I felt completely fine. Parents were asked to leave the room so the children could acclimatise in the classroom on their own and I too felt relaxed about leaving him as he played on the class computer and didn't even look up as I left. That was until I saw another tiny girl being peeled off her daddy in floods of tears and that set me off snivelling! It wasn't even about my own child! Zac was cool and didn't even look up and there I was filling up about someone else's baby starting school!

The timing of Zac leaving nursery and starting school, coupled with our recent failed cycle of IVF, made the fact that we didn't have another baby all the more obvious. The void felt like it was even greater and as the chapters of Zac's life seemed to be zooming along, I really felt the pain of other chapters not starting all the more during that summer.

One day in the office when Dom was ribbing me about being soft about Zac starting school, I could feel my anxiety building in my chest as I struggled to contain my emotions. We would often pull each other's leg about things and normally I would laugh along with him but I just couldn't find it in me to laugh about this. I just wanted to scream at him and tell him it wasn't just that Zac was starting school, it was that my time with nursery was ending. My baby time would be finished, gone, never to be repeated. I had a child now. A schoolboy. Not a little boy, not a baby and that chapter was now ended when I didn't want it to. I couldn't keep Zac at nursery of course, but I still wanted to need their services, wanted that chapter to stay open, and wanted to be a mummy to a baby once more.

Buying his uniform and shopping for shoes wasn't as exciting as I had always hoped it might be. It felt like every move towards the start of term in September was painful and I was dragging my feet trying to slow the calendar down. The timing was painful and torturous.

I had the feeling that I wanted to just escape from it all and we agreed a holiday would help. I wanted to go as soon as possible in June but it was impossible with my work commitments and the only possible week I was able to go was my birthday week at the end of July. We booked an all inclusive hotel in Majorca and the thought of doing nothing for a week seemed just what Jason and I needed. We had a fun week and I'll always remember watching the Olympics with Zac each day during that holiday. He loved learning all about the new sports he'd never seen before and learning about new heroes such as Usain Bolt, Mo Farah and David Weir.

The timing of the holiday was perfect actually as it was around the time the first pregnancy would have been due. I didn't get hung up on a specific date, as I knew Zac had been 3 weeks early, but the month of July had been looming with some meaning for a while. It had been my first 'due date', my first cycle, first and only positive pregnancy test. Now, here we were able to go on a holiday to Spain because it was just the three of us still. No newborn. No new baby goodies packed in the suitcase, in fact no new life with the bigger family I thought we were destined for.

The significance hadn't escaped me. We spoke about it briefly but both felt we needed to brush it aside just as quickly because, as ever, the pain and negativity was just too much. In a way we weren't dealing with it, but on the other hand, our way of dealing with our future going forward was to focus ahead and not dwell on what we couldn't change behind us.

July was also significant as it was my birthday. Another birthday, another milestone, another bloody year older. I turned 39 when we were in Spain and whilst I had a fabulous meal out on the marina with my boys, the knowledge that my chances of conceiving got slimmer that day made my celebrations bittersweet. The boys did all they could to make my day special and I will never, ever forget the gorgeous gift Jason surprised me with. He and Zac proudly gave me a box to open and inside was the most gorgeous diamond pendant. I was totally shocked! It was stunning. Jason explained how he knew I'd been through a lot and was really low but that he and Zac wanted to show how much they loved me and appreciated what I'd done for them. To this day, the thought of their gesture overwhelms me. Of course, what girl wouldn't love a diamond pendant? But to me, whilst it was beautiful and obviously cost a lot of money, it was more the fact that Jason had thought to buy me such a super special gift and given it to me with such meaning that made that present so precious. I had never had, and probably will never again, such an amazing gift, both in terms of 'wow' and meaning!

It was a solitaire with eight tiny diamonds round the outside. It was given to me because of everything I'd been through that last year. We'd had three cycles but four embryos that sadly didn't stay with me, so I felt it was two diamonds for each and one large one for Zac to look after them. I immediately felt a huge attachment to the necklace and my lost embies. As well as beautiful, I found the necklace so healing, such a positive focus and to this day I squeeze the pendant when I remember what we lost. It will always be an incredibly sentimental necklace. A few weeks later a friend remarked "oh so it's not just one solitaire?" almost as if it were a cheap imitation and yet the comment didn't sting as much as it might have done, had the eight diamonds round the small solitaire not had such a huge meaning. "No" I replied confidently. "That's right."

We had thought about taking my Mum on the holiday with us but had decided that we needed time as a couple on our own to talk things through about our options and next steps. This turned out to be the best and worst decision. It was for the best as the hotel complex was enormous with thousands of steps which Mum simply wouldn't have been able to cope with, but it was also the worst decision as Zac demanded 100% of our time. As it turned out we had very little time to talk.

When we did manage to grab some thinking time alone and then time to chat things through together, we both decided that we weren't done yet. We considered the huge investment we'd already made and calculated how much more we would need to go through it again. It was a huge gamble and the treatment was eating into everything we had. We knew we couldn't go on forever and that there would little left if we did go again. Yet neither of us felt ready to give up and we both did feel we had the strength to try again. We were both unsure about what the future would hold if we stepped onto that path once more and agreed that we needed the appointment from the clinic to know if it was possible, feasible or advisable to continue. One thing that was clear though, was that both of us felt able to continue, didn't feel like we'd finished and the fact that we both came to that conclusion independently gave us the strength to pursue the next step which would be to see whether the experts thought the same. We wanted to take the risk.

I made one firm decision on that holiday and that was that I wasn't going to start anything until after my brother's wedding. I had missed out on so much the previous year or been at events where I had felt shocking. I was determined not to spoil such a fantastic family occasion. I wanted to focus

100% on my brother and Kate, I wanted to enjoy the day for what it was and not be distracted or preoccupied with wanting a baby in any way. Most of all I wanted to feel well, to have a drink if I felt like it and to feel special in my bridesmaid dress. I'd spend months feeling like a bloated whale, in pain and in clothes that were then too tight and I was adamant that I wasn't going to feel that way on their big day. I had of course wanted to be as big as a whale and had envisaged having a huge bump under my bridesmaid dress so now, as that wasn't going to be the case, I wanted to forget all the treatment and enjoy a special day. That definite decision helped my sanity at that time in the summer. Just like after the first cycle when Zac's birthday party helped me focus on something different, making a decision not to do anything at all helped me to relax in the weeks in the run up to the big day.

I knew Debbie would be pregnant. I also knew from the dates I'd calculated for my own would-be pregnancy that she would be coming up to 12 weeks and a few weeks before the wedding I asked Mum if she'd heard. She said yes she thought she was, as she'd been told she was, but not heard any more. It was the strangest answer when a yes or no would have sufficed and though I was aware I had caught mum off guard and she obviously felt bad at being the one to tell me, it was a bitter pill lacking any sugar in the way it was delivered. It hit me full on in the stomach. Yes, she said yes, so yes, she is pregnant. She is pregnant, it did work, and she's having a baby. Her treatment was successful. That is what Mum's garbled response actually meant.

I hate the human mind for the crazy mixed up feelings it throws up for us, but I guess it was all to be expected. I was really so pleased that she was expecting and particularly that my little cousin wouldn't have to go through any more heartache or any more treatments. I was also thrilled because for as long as I can remember, Debbie has always been maternal and been great with her nieces and nephew. And yet, as expected, as we would have been sharing the same due dates and pregnancy milestones and if I'm honest as it was my third time and only her first, I was absolutely gutted. Why? There was no answer, no justification. Mum called and confirmed a few days later that she was definitely pregnant, as she'd seen a scan photo on Facebook. This time I was more pleased, my own initial disappointment now subsiding. It still felt so strange though to know someone else's exact milestone dates for their pregnancy. I knew how many weeks she'd be at Andrew's wedding; how far at Christmas and the week she would be due. They had been my dates too for a while.

Days and weeks flew by and the time soon came for Zac's Nursery leaving party that was an annual fun day event attended by all the families from the entire nursery. I had been dreading it though Zac expressed great excitement, as he knew all the children were presented with a special teddy bear and cuddle from Sally. The families of the leavers had all pulled together and presented the team with a brand new dressing up wardrobe as a leaving gift. It was so sad to say goodbye to his friends and their families, some of whom were going on to different primary schools. It was the end of an era; the end of what had felt like a really close-knit group and it was a very emotional day. It was so sad to leave the team for the last time as each of them gave Zac a hug and you could see that they all loved that little man so much.

A few days before, whilst at work, the nursery team had sent me a photograph of Zac and his friend outside the local pub at lunchtime as Sally and her family had taken them their for a special treat to celebrate them leaving. They all still had the Olympics bug and were doing Mo Farah's 'Mobot' stance outside the front door. It was another reminder of how lucky I was to have such a wonderful child who was so obviously loved by so many other people, and caused me to question why I was putting myself through hell and back with IVF treatment for another child when actually I was so blessed already. What was I thinking? On his final day, Zac with his best friends, Harry and Eva all gave a special gift to their key worker Sam and had photos as the three of them gave her extra hugs. We would miss her so much, they adored her and she adored them just as much. We waved as we walked to the car, waved from the car and as we honked the horn down the driveway, all the staff came out on the steps and waved us off. I was crying my eyes out. It really was over. Zac had left nursery, but moreover, so had I.

That summer many of my girlfriends were turning 40 so we enjoyed plenty of parties and trips away. As we were in a position where we couldn't do anything to help us conceive other than continue to have sex, it was a strangely nice period where Jason and I didn't have to talk about it. It was like the huge elephant in the room was wearing a disguise momentarily, he was still there we just couldn't see him right now!

I had a few drinks to enjoy each occasion but didn't go mad and continued with my healthy eating of super foods, cutting out caffeine and plenty of training with Duncan and Zumba. I was feeling great in myself, my arms were toned and my abs were really starting to tone up too. Having spent months feeling bloated, it was really refreshing to feel positive about my body and show it off a bit more, which I hadn't felt like doing in months. I was still mindful that I needed to keep my body the best it could be in case we could proceed with more treatment and I was enjoying looking after myself.

I went on a girl's trip to Portugal to celebrate three of my friends' 40th birthdays. We stayed in a villa, sharing rooms and from the moment I left our house, I was up for having a good time and enjoying myself. This was a trip I hadn't planned on going on and I'd previously declined thinking I'd be pregnant, so now, especially with no immediate plans for treatment, there was nothing to stop me from letting my hair down. Sun, gossip, great company and an introduction to passion fruit mojitos should have been the perfect combination for a relaxing and fun few days.

I was feeling good in myself, feeling fit and healthy and had bought some nice new clothes and bikinis so was feeling better than I had in ages. My heart was still heavy and my emotions subdued but I was determined to try to enjoy the moment.

On the first full day, we were by the pool and I was telling the girls about how terrific I thought Julie's Zumba class was. After not being able to persuade Jules to do a class for us on the lawn, I attempted to show the girls some of her moves. I did them no justice at all and I'm sure Julie was desperate for me to sit down and shut up, but we were all laughing so much and it felt great to laugh. As I sat back down and took another slurp of my drink to recover, a few of the girls commented on my toned tummy and how good it looked when I was doing the moves. I started to explain how I had been working out and focussing on my stomach to hopefully prepare for pregnancy. It felt OK to talk about it and I didn't feel upset.

A couple of hours later, I was still relaxing by the pool, with one of my friends I don't see as often as the other girls. She put her hand on mine and said she knew she hadn't spoken to me much about my treatment but that some of the others had kept her updated and that I should know she was always thinking of me. She asked me a few questions and I slowly began to open up and talk about the last failed cycle. The relaxing in the sun, probably the drink and now being with someone being nice to me, were undoubtedly the worst combination for someone trying to be strong and brave about something. I started crying. That familiar involuntary drip of tears.

A couple of the girls came over but I tried to shrug them off and pull myself together. I was on a fun girls trip away, I couldn't cry, didn't want to spoil it with my depressive mood. And yet it was increasingly hard to hide my sadness. It felt like a big, heavy, dark cape I was wearing. It had taken my appetite, my enjoyment of the usual Portuguese treats I so loved and my enthusiasm for the silly games and trivia the girls were playing. It was suppressing me and I longed for it to be lifted. Try as I might I couldn't shake off my deepest sadness and I was struggling to cover it up when we were in such relaxing surroundings. So, I cried and I talked and I let them all in a little on why it was so hard this time and how desperately sad I felt right now and then I cried some more.

In fact at various intervals for the rest of the trip I found myself either crying fully or fighting back tears. The numbness was starting to lift and the pain of the previous few months that had been bottling up was now starting to leak out. It was a shock to me that I should be crying again and it was a scary prospect that I was starting to have to deal with something that I was terrified of.

It was all very well feeling and looking good on the outside, but behind the tight abs and sun kissed face was a broken girl. A girl struggling to smile, to laugh, to hold a conversation without blurting out "I'm not pregnant!" For once in my life I didn't care that the girls were complimenting me on my figure or that I felt confident in my short dresses because I just felt beaten. Completely overpowered by the emotional strain of not just three cycles not working but by the fear that this might always be the case and there was nothing I could do to change it. As if my body had gone into battle but lost. It looked great but it didn't work. I hated myself and I for a moment I hated everyone there for not seeing beyond my tight tummy. None of that fucking mattered if I felt such sadness beyond belief inside.

And yet I also loved those girls during those few days. Not knowing how to really help my situation, they let me cry, let me talk, let me be silent if I wanted but most of all they made me laugh! They got up to such crazy, stupid antics that it was impossible not to laugh and it was a terrific tonic for me. I returned home tanned, with some great memories and a little lighter from actually having cried openly for the first time in ages.

Preparing to try again

September was now fully upon us and Zac was starting school. Swamped in his new uniform we proudly took photographs of him on the lawn, holding his new book bag, all ready to set off on his first day. The school seemed huge and he seemed tiny, and that was just how I felt about it, so heaven knows how my little fella felt himself.

This was a huge milestone for both of us and now, being a full time working Mum, the enormity of a full time job and having a child at school were all starting to hit me. Nursery was so much easier as we could drop him off and collect him either side of our working hours but with Zac now finishing at 3.30pm and having school holidays, it was placing increasing pressure on Jason and I. We booked him a place in after-school club and decided that between us, we would take him ourselves in the morning. I had always got to the office just after nine anyway and after all, I had started working for myself so that I could have options like this open to me. I already had family commitments and I was always clear I wanted to extend the family. It was exactly times like these where I could fully take advantage of my fortunate position.

Zac starting school was such a massive deal for me and as the day drew nearer it was far greater than I, and definitely anyone else, could have imagined. The thought that he might be the only child I would ever have was increasingly bearing heavy on my mind. I simply couldn't shake it off that this might be my one and only experience of my child starting school, of them holding my hand as we walked into the playground and of my tiny child, who looked so small at the top of the school steps, running towards me at home time. I wanted to slow down the clocks, savour every minute and ensure I gave Zac everything I had and that he could want. That meant me, my time, my attention and as smooth a transition to him starting school as possible. So, whilst we booked him into after-school club, I also decided that I would collect him from school on a Monday and Friday at 3.30pm and then work from home. I didn't want to miss seeing him go in through the doors in the morning and I didn't want to miss seeing his delighted little face at the top of the steps, when he saw my face in the sea of other parents at the end of each day. If this was to be my only child then I didn't want to miss out on anything. I felt more comfortable once I decided to do this and Zac was definitely happy with the arrangement.

Dom questioned my arrangement when I initially told him and Emma and said his kids were fine in the after school club and that Zac would be fine there also. I knew Zac would be fine, just as I knew his boys were, but it was about so much more than simply the quality of childcare for me. I worked for myself, I could easily get my work done at home after collecting him and I felt that as I was fortunate to have the choice, I wanted to collect him myself. At that time I felt more than ever that children were such a gift that you should look after them, give them all you can and cherish every minute as they grow up so quickly. Where had the last four and a half years gone for starters? I felt I had already missed out on so much with Zac, taken for granted there would be other children that would remind me of the various stages of growing up and right now, I wasn't prepared to miss a single second of my boy. I knew my business partners weren't wholly happy with my decision and yet as it turned out I often got more work done in the two or three hours I worked at home after collecting him. Being flexible in working environment wasn't something we had really come across before, except if the boiler man was calling at home or we were poorly and yet to me, I knew I would get my work done and I didn't see it as the problem that they did. Understandably their view of the world was completely different to mine at that time. The business was their main priority and as much as I cared and as hard as I worked, I had an enormous distraction in my life and my priorities were now different to theirs. It was understandable they would have concerns of course, but with all this, I fell a little bit out of love with my own business.

The arrival of September also meant Andrew and Kate's wedding and it was one of the most enjoyable family days I can ever remember. I was so proud of what they pulled off. Kate simply looked stunning. She took my breath away and seeing her and Andrew together I couldn't believe our luck that he had found such a wonderful person to share his life with and welcome into our family. Mum looked amazing and it was nice to see her amongst friends as the centre of attention and feeling great for a change. Minnie was a super cute flower girl. Jason, as ever, looked dapper and I loved my family so much that day I was on cloud nine.

Zac was a pageboy, or 'Captain Usher' as he and Andrew preferred to call him, and he looked so grown up and gorgeous in an outfit matching the groom and ushers that also included a proud Daddy. The only slight complication was that Zac hated trousers. He hadn't worn long pants for almost eighteen months in fact, in January he had been on Filey beach in wellies, hat, scarf, gloves and shorts! He absolutely hated long pants and used to complain that the fabric tickled his legs. When trying on his outfit in the Men's outfitters he'd been excited and really pleased to be wearing the same as Daddy and Uncle Andrew. Yet on the morning, with Jason who was getting him ready on his own, Zac had thrown several tantrums refusing to wear the trousers! I'm not sure how he was persuaded in the end but I do know from looking at all the photographs that he wasn't happy about it at all. He was pouting and looking grumpy in every single shot! So hilarious! The only photos of Zac smiling on the day were at the reception when he was allowed to put his shorts on and kick an inflatable football around the dance floor! Yet, I couldn't have been prouder of my boy.

As I came out of church, hugging and kissing my many aunts, uncles and cousins, I saw Debbie. I felt weak, nervous even shy. I loved the girl, she was my flesh and blood, my family so how could I possibly be feeling like this? I'd had butterflies for days before wondering how I'd be when I came face to face with her. I also hated myself for even questioning that I might not just simply be happy to see her and congratulate her on her news. Why did my evil, jealous, pained thoughts have to enter my head at all?

It was a strange mix of feelings as I really was so thrilled for her but I felt sick when I first saw her and her tiny bump. That tummy flip was fleeting though and I hugged and congratulated her and her partner at their wonderful news. Once I had done that I felt better instantly. It had been such a big deal to see her even though I knew whether she got pregnant or not had no bearing on whether I would conceive again. She was expecting another addition to our family, I loved her dearly and I was now excited for her.

My size 12 dress obviously had to be taken in all over and was now somewhat slightly misshapen when compared to Kate's sister Elaine's dress but I felt lovely none-the-less. It was perhaps ironic that the other bridesmaid,

Kate's best friend Rachel, actually ended up having a different style dress to us altogether as she was six months pregnant and had a huge bump up front. So a bump did follow Kate down the aisle afterall, it just wasn't mine.

I couldn't believe it! We had all been dress shopping together and myself and Elaine had certain frocks we liked turned down because Rachel didn't think they'd flatter her shape, when all the time, we were all unaware that she was newly expecting! Once again I reminded myself that someone else's good fortune did not deny me my pregnancy but, once again, the timing was incredible. That bump is in the wrong dress, on the wrong person! I was supposed to be the huge bridesmaid! That was my dream, my desire but sadly not my reality. Of course I was pleased for Rachel, who was a delightful girl and fab Mummy already, but it was crushing for me that day. If I was not to have a baby for Andrew's wedding I felt certain I would at least have a bump, large or small, I hadn't cared. I was not supposed to be in a dress a size too big, that had been taken in all over, to the extent that it was now almost a completely different design, to accommodate my flat, empty tummy and normal sized boobs!... I could have ranted, could have been upset, but there was so much love and joy it was a tonic to focus on what Andrew and Kate had created. It was an amazing day and I loved them both so much for what they had achieved together.

Later that night, a few Bacardi and Cokes later, it was time to go home and so began the lengthy goodbyes to all the family. A couple of my aunties who had known about our recent failed cycle, held and hugged me for a little longer. Their overwhelming love burst my floodgates. Huge, drunken sobs shook me in my misshapen dress. I was tired, tipsy and if I was honest, touched by their love and kindness towards me. It was hard, it did hurt and it just wasn't supposed to be that way. I hated feeling that I should be a person that required sympathy. I heard "I'm so sorry" and whilst I knew they were and knew they loved me, it never felt easy hearing someone say that to me. In a way it made the sorry situation more of a reality. God it hurt so much that night.

Dare we go for a fourth attempt?

It was October and as I'm not very good at being dishonest or keeping secrets and as they were my business partners after all, I told Emma and Dom that I was thinking of having another go but we needed to see the Prof at our next appointment to determine if and when we could go for it. There was little they could say to this, although they said they expected it to be the following year and presumed I would be leaving the treatment until after Christmas. I felt guilty for saying that I genuinely didn't know when our appointment would come through but that I thought it would probably be sooner than that.

I felt awkward and cornered and angry for feeling that way. To them, I know, it was important and I had used all my holiday for treatment that year previously but to me, nothing else was important and I was alarmed at their initial response, but then angered by their second. "You know you've not got any holidays left." I had already worked out my holiday allocation and so was prepared to say I'd take the week off unpaid, but I hadn't been prepared to be discussing it at this early stage. We hadn't even had the meeting yet, we didn't even know if we would be able to have a fourth attempt. The more I was getting involved with the treatment that year, the more my views on life were becoming further and further away from those around me. They were wholly supportive but there were moments where their priorities and concerns were poles apart from mine and in my hyper-sensitive state, I found this really difficult to deal with at times. I was trying to be open, honest and practical about what was on my mind and I guess, from their perspective, so were they.

Later that week a management meeting was called to decide if we were trying to run a profitable business or a lifestyle business. I knew the question was directed at myself and when I pressed my partners, they admitted they weren't happy about my time collecting Zac on a Monday and Friday and wanted to know how long I was planning on continuing to pick him up. There comes times in life when some things that were really important to you, suddenly don't seem important any longer. Again, I fell out of love with my own business a little more that day and it was upsetting. I set up working for myself to help fit around my family's lifestyle and I knew that with my talent and experience there was no reason why it shouldn't be profitable also. I said as much and also expressed that I thought it was why we'd all set up together. Why couldn't it be both? I was somewhat torn between being really hurt and not giving a stuff. I was already an animal with a wound I was trying to deal with, but now to be dealt a second blow challenging my time with my son and a further blow questioning my input to the business when working from home. It really, really stung. We all had different lives, different lifestyles, different ways we took advantage of our working circumstances and yet I was being questioned about mine. More than anything I felt there was little trust and I think it was this that hurt more than anything.

To my mind, I had pulled myself in so many different directions over the last year, but I had always tried to put in 100% when it came to the business. Yes I'd used my holidays for treatment days and yet I'd sat at my desk at times feeling horrendous, but I'd never let anything drop or let anyone down and now to be challenged I felt like I was the one being let down. Looking back, I know it had been a tough 12 months affecting everyone around me and I can only imagine the circus that I must have created each time I went through the treatment. Here I was, about to start all over again, so it was probably natural for them to want to know what it would mean for them. I'm sure they would both have longed for a partner who was settled and without complication, but I also hope we all learned something about working for yourself that day, in that you can have it all, a work/lifestyle balance and profit, if you just give it your all and trust each other.

I was feeling weak and vulnerable however. I had kept all my emotions in a box for so long and now, contemplating the possibility of another round, they were all starting to surface. Other than brief conversations in Portugal, I'd not spoken, not really cried very much and not dealt with my grief fully. A couple of times I'd called the clinic for the counsellor's number but then felt foolish, so never called. I actually once got as far as receiving an application form for counselling but again, didn't know what I would say other than "I'm not pregnant and it's making me sad" so I ripped it up and forgot about any plans to go and talk to someone.

A week or two later, one of Zac's nursery friends was having a birthday party and it was great to see lots of familiar faces again, amongst the parents as well as the children. As the children tucked into their tea, I started talking to one of the mums next to me, who I recognised but only from passing in the nursery car park at drop off. It was then that I met someone who was to become an exceptionally close friend in the future. Bizarrely, as conversations go sometimes, we immediately clicked and were talking about all sorts of personal information, swapping stories and experiences and it was then that she asked me if I just had Zac or whether I had any other children. Pausing, in a split second I thought about how to answer, but surprisingly heard myself say that we would love another child and were about to have our fourth round of IVF. Well I was confident at least! We hadn't actually agreed we would or indeed been told by the clinic that we could or should, but it appeared I was believing that we going to give it a go!

Strangely we had something in common. She too was struggling to have a second child and was considering IVF treatment. I immediately offered support, advice and answered the barrage of questions that she threw at me. She had no idea about anything to do with the treatment at that stage, she hadn't read anything and she was frightened about the prospect of embarking on that path. I really felt like I knew exactly where she was in fact; she was exactly where I had been just twelve months before. Staring at the only route that seemed open, staring into the unknown. Desperate for answers, yet struggling to know what questions to even ask. After the party, we were thrown out of the play centre but spent a further hour talking in the car park, whilst our boys played in and out of the hedgerows.

We kept in touch via email and as she was reading up on the subject I was answering more and more questions and it was nice to feel I was able to pass on the knowledge to help someone else, just as Jo had always been there for me.

And yet, there was a large part of me that wanted to back off, not get too involved. By now we had received our appointment date from the clinic and I was starting to look forward and think about our next attempt. She too had received a date from the clinic and I was quickly becoming worried about getting hurt again. I didn't want to follow someone else's journey only to be disappointed by their success and my failure. I couldn't cope with the stress and strain of following anyone else's treatment again, like Debbie, as I was struggling to muster the strength to support myself. We continued to chat via emails but I really had the feeling that I needed to be selfish and look after myself so tried as hard as I could not to get overly involved. A few times I talked to my Mum about how I was wrestling with my feelings. I was really keen to support her and help her and yet I knew I hardly had enough strength to get myself through the treatment, let alone anyone else. I simply couldn't risk any additional hurt again. I knew I needed to be selfish but it wasn't my natural instinct. As hard as it would be in forthcoming weeks, I needed to keep my distance, just simply for self-preservation.

In deciding to try once more, I hadn't approached the attempt in the same way as I had before. I was still flat, still emotionless, still absolutely devastated by the failure of the third attempt. I knew I hadn't dealt with it or grieved properly and certainly hadn't picked myself up in a way I would have previously tried to in the past.

I had once totally believed that a positive spirit and 'can do' attitude would be a huge part of being successful in anything and to have been proven wrong was something I was still trying to come to terms with. I was running on empty and still felt completely broken by the whole process. My attitude this time was so unlike anything I had experienced before that it was difficult to recognise my thoughts as my own. I felt that I was still so down and shattered by the last year, that at least if we tried and failed this time, it wouldn't hurt as much as I hadn't picked myself up from the last time. I really believed that building myself up to approach the treatment feeling positive, was the worst thing I could do at that time and anyway, I had done that last time and it had been proved to be completely futile, so what was the point? At least this time, we were starting from rock bottom so there wasn't as far to fall.

When our appointment finally came round to meet Professor Killick, my mood was still low and I arrived at the clinic feeling strangely numb once more. The usual churned up cocktail of excitement and apprehension was masked with a quiet, nonchalant numbness that meant I was perhaps strangely without conversation for once. I had really low expectations and for the first time I felt there was little hope that we would be able to have another go, let alone be successful. If I'm honest, I was probably also terrified that they might turn round and say there was no point trying again, and there was a real possibility that they may indeed do that. The one in three chance statistics kept going round and round in my head. We'd had three chances and failed, was there any point trying again?

I was to be pleasantly surprised. After going through our very thick file, cycle by cycle and asking us various questions about each element of each attempt, Prof concluded by saying: "I would love to tell you that you should stop, grieve, enjoy Zac and get on with your life but I don't really think that and the file doesn't tell me that."

Instantly hope began to flicker a little within me. So, he's saying we can go again? I'll never forget his words and analogies as he went on: "To have a one in three chance you need to roll a three sided dice four times. You've rolled it three times and got a one, and three and then three again. You've landed on three twice and you need to roll again to have a chance of getting that two!" It kind of sort of made sense, even though it didn't, but it was enough to start to get me excited.

We talked about my reaction to the drugs, the hyper-stimulation and how poorly I had been both times at the fresh transfers. Prof then said: "To take a perfect photograph you go towards the cliff edge and go as far as you possibly can to get the best possible view. If you go too far, you fall off and get no picture at all, so you have to work out the perfect place to stand to get the perfect picture. In your case, we have taken you too far each time and we need to approach with great caution this time." Again, it sort of made sense.

It was starting to sink in that he might be saying we could have another go and that we still had a chance of success but I desperately wanted to know I wasn't being foolish in wanting to try again. I asked him directly: "Prof, I'm the sort of person that if you tell me I can't climb a tree, I'll have a bloody good go to show you that I can, whether I can or not. We so desperately want another child that I will just keep going and going with IVF trying to have one as long as I can, so if there is *anything* in the file or anything that makes you think that we might not be successful then I *need* you to tell me to stop. I know I won't stop myself. I need someone to tell me and force me to stop. I don't want to keep going and keep trying when everyone around me thinks I'm foolish because they don't think it will work. I have a kid who needs his Mummy so if there is any part of you that thinks I should, then I'm begging you to tell me to stop today."

I knew I was crying uncontrollably. I'd lost it. I'd used the word begging and as strong a word as that was, I'd meant it. I almost wanted him to stand me up and grab me by both arms, shake me and shout, "stop, stop, just stop, it's no use." This part of our meeting was so important. It was vital for my sanity. The last 12 months had taken so much out of both of us and we could easily be blinded by our desire for another child, that we could have ignored the effect it was having on us, on Zac and on everyone around us. At that time it seemed there was only one thing important to me and I would stop at nothing to get it, so I needed to know there and then if there was any reason we should stop trying. If there was, then we needed to stop and as Prof said, grieve, get back to giving Zac 100% and move on enjoying life as a family of three. Stop chasing tomorrow's dream at the cost of today's happiness. But I couldn't stop it myself. I needed Prof to get hold of me and insist I stop. He would have to tell me.

But he put the file down, sat back in his chair and smiled in a way I knew and hoped he'd smiled at thousands of couples before. It was his smile that said 'I still think there is hope.' What he actually said was: "I think you've just been unlucky so far. There is no reason why you shouldn't be pregnant, I honestly think you've just had bad luck."

I was somewhat shocked, stunned but hugely relieved. It felt like the clouds parted and a tiny chink of light, one bright ray of sunshine lit up the room. I literally felt a heavy weight lift from somewhere deep within me. I'd really not expected such a positive response and everything he said really made sense to our situation.

We discussed the OHSS and he suggested the slowest dose of stimulation and the introduction of a new drug, Metformin that would hopefully improve the quality of eggs produced so that we would go for quality over quantity. We discussed the bleeding each time after a week following the two fresh cycles and he suggested injections instead of pessaries, which was music to my ears. Who knew they did injections? I hated those bloody pessaries so much that this bit of news alone made me feel elated!

It felt really positive that having considered our case in great detail and learned from the past three cycles, he had offered us alternative routes forward. They were only small tweaks and had no guarantee but overall we had hope again, we had a new plan, a new set of drugs and we felt it was right to go again. There was also no reason to delay or to wait any longer. We felt utterly liberated and I really felt that the weight of potentially feeling foolish and that others might doubt us, had finally been lifted. We could have another go, we should have another go and we still had a good chance of success.

We received a letter shortly afterwards confirming the details and we sent a cheque off for the drugs and treatment. All we had to do now was wait for my period and get our heads round the fact that we were going again!

A different approach

It was a strange feeling embarking on the fourth cycle, in a way it almost didn't feel like we were really doing it at all. Previously it had been such a huge part of our lives and our conversation but this time, it was just something we'd be doing over the next few weeks and life went on as normal.

I still felt so low and upset from the last three, and in particular the third attempt, that I didn't have the strength to muster to get into a positive frame of mind. I was still eating healthily and exercising but I was approaching it more aggressively in a weird way. I was now doing those things because I wanted to, not because I had to.

It almost felt like my mood couldn't possibly get any lower and my spirit be any more broken, so we may as well have another go. At least this time the fall wouldn't be so great if we failed and the pain not as severe. 'Bring it on' was my attitude. 'Come and try to hurt me because it's impossible to hurt me more than I am now!' 'Have a go, do your worst, try your hardest, but you can't make this pain any greater!'

It sounds crazy to go again when I obviously hadn't grieved from the last time, but I was becoming harder, putting walls up to protect myself and it was the only way I could even think about getting through another round. If I had taken time out, grieved, pulled myself through and started to rebuild to feel positive for another round, I honestly think it would have finished me off. Dealing with the hurt, the grief, the pain, the worry, was just not an option. I had to go now, or never at all. I guess it brought out the fight in me.

My view was definitely that the best way not to get hurt was to not fix myself, not build myself up, not be optimistic, just go through the motions as we were now doing and see what happened.

I started to feel that I couldn't bear any more attempts so I may as well have another go whilst I was feeling so low and avoid the huge blow that any failure could have brought in the future.

The date came through for my drug collection and receipt of the new plan so I went during my lunchtime and heading up to reception where I once again cheerily said "Hi" to the girls. As I paid for the drugs and treatment, I glanced down the invoice and noticed the Utrogestan pessaries were on the bill when the Prof had said we were switching to the injections. I mentioned it to the receptionist who then mentioned it to Debbie the nurse. I explained the changes to the plan that Prof had mentioned as we went through all the drugs on the invoice. I questioned the Utrogestan and then noticed that the Metformin was missing, as were the injections. Debbie seemed confused as she said they hadn't used those injections for more than two years.

It seemed I was being given the same plan and drugs as the last two fresh cycles with no changes or any amended plan designed specifically for me! I started crying. It had been a big deal to get my head around going through this again and apart from still wanting another baby, the only reason I was doing this, was the hope that Prof had given us and the thought that these slight changes to the plan might help us.

I was in total shock. I instantly felt that they had taken away my hope, my plan, and the reason we decided to go ahead again. Everything Prof had suggested had been ignored and was now being questioned. The last time we were in the clinic we started to feel like we were getting somewhere and now, just days later, I was immediately starting to lose confidence and crumble all over again.

Debbie said she'd go and try to find Prof but returned moments later saying he was lecturing but that she would take down all my queries and speak to him later that afternoon. They told me to go with the bag of drugs I had and start the injections that night, as any changes wouldn't make any difference to the first injections anyway.

"It looks like we don't know what we're doing!" she said trying to lighten my mood and make me laugh as she had successfully done so often before. I wanted to say, "yes it does" but didn't. As she was talking she was flicking through my file saying that she'd finally found a copy of Prof's letter to us but also had the audit meeting notes which stated to stick to the same plan as before.

I went back to the reception desk and tapped my pin number in to pay. Unusually for me I didn't look up to the girls, didn't chat, didn't flash a smile or a joke and clearly noting my demeanour, Roxanne asked if I was all right. I burst into tears yet still didn't lift my head as I explained that "Prof's changes to our treatment had given us the hope that it might work this time and now not only had they given us different drugs but they couldn't agree on a plan and it's not what I was expecting and I'm just in shock" – or something to that effect as I know I was rambling in between my heavy sobs and sniffles. I assured them I was OK, not to worry and tried to muster a smile before I took my credit card, turned and hurried towards the door.

Climbing into the car in the car park, I sat in the chair with the huge brown paper bag of drugs on my knee staring down at the many boxes of drugs. I felt in a state of shock. I didn't know whether I should call and tell Jason or just leave it, go back to work and wait until I heard from the clinic later that afternoon.

I was supposed to be starting my first injection that night! Today was the start of our fourth round and increasingly it was starting to feel like our final round and last chance. And yet it didn't seem like anybody was in control of what I'd be taking. Nobody could agree on what would be the best way forward. How could I start on this journey, putting these drugs inside me when we're not sure we've got a plan that is going to work and the team don't seem to know what they're on about?

Apart from what this could potentially mean at the end of the treatment this was the last of my hard fought for life savings in this bloody bag! This was perhaps new clothes for Zac, day trips, holidays, repairs to the house and so on! It was a bloody lot of money to be spending that I certainly didn't want to feel we were wasting!

I grew increasingly agitated and anxious in the car as I stared at the bag of drugs then back at the hospital building and back to the drugs again. If I was going to start another round I wanted to do so in the knowledge that we had the very best chance of it working. I didn't feel that way. I didn't feel in the least bit confident and I couldn't afford financially or emotionally to enter into this without feeling 100% certain that it was the right thing to do. I didn't think it would work but I still wanted to get to the other end knowing that at least I had done everything I could and I really believed that learning from past cycles and changing the drugs made some sense. I was about to spend £4,000 and inject myself with drugs when I wasn't sure we'd got the best plan that would give the best chance. I must be mad! Well no, I wasn't mad and I wasn't stupid enough to do so, but I was angry. In fact, by now I was furious, like a woman possessed!

What happened next was almost autopilot and a behaviour I had never experienced before, literally never, ever in my life experienced before! I rarely lose control or composure but as I locked the car and marched towards the hospital, carrying my bag of drugs, I could feel something taking over my once broken body, making me feel strong and fearless. It was like something else was operating my body and voice. I've lost my temper but this was another level! This was something else and it was frightening!

I was going over and over my thoughts as I made my way with gusto back to the clinic. There was simply no way I could start the bloody treatment when doubting that it might work. I couldn't do it to myself but moreover I couldn't put Zac, my family or friends through it either. It wasn't fair.

This was it, this felt like the final chance and if I was to start with this cycle then I needed to start that night and I was in no way confident that I would be taking the right drugs. So they either made me confident, switched the drugs or we abandoned the cycle until next time. Either way, I needed answers and I needed them now, not later in the day.

I was panting both with exertion and anger as I reached the door and pressed the buzzer. Letting me in, Roxanne immediately came round from behind reception straight over to me saying they had all been really worried about me.

"I need to see a consultant Roxanne please, and I need to see them today, in fact now." I was angry, I was breathless but I also wanted to try to retain my composure as I had almost lost it marching from the car.

Roxanne headed towards the treatment rooms where Debbie and Caroline quickly came out to see me. We all sat down in the waiting room, which was fortunately empty of people, and they tried to calm me down. I explained how I was feeling, what the Prof had said, why we had decided to try again and why now I had completely lost all confidence and didn't know whether it was right to proceed or not.

The girls tried to console me and calm me down and said "We hate to see you like this Helen." I stood up then, anger returning. Looking them in the eye and starting to lose the composure I had worked so hard to retain I whispered loudly through my snotty tears. "But this IS me! This is the *real* me! This is what you don't see, this is what it's like, what this place makes you like! Behind my laughs and smiles and jokes, this is what is going on inside me, day in, day out. I *hate* being like this, but this is it, this IS ME!"

They looked slightly alarmed but I'm sure had seen girls like this before and I'm sure far worse. They tried to get me to sit down but I was pacing the floor up and down by now. I couldn't sit down. I just couldn't keep still. They agreed to send someone to find Prof and get him out of his lecture. I'm usually quite obliging and would never normally put anyone to any trouble, but right then and there I didn't care who was inconvenienced, I couldn't go home with my plan in question and a bag of drugs nobody could agree on.

The nurses returned to the treatment room and Roxanne returned to her desk behind the reception glass screen while I waited for Prof to arrive. I was alone, but I couldn't stop pacing the floor. It all kept going over and over in my head. My anger, my upset, my frustration and by this stage my surprise at my apparent behaviour! What on earth had come over me to come out with an outburst like that?

Prof came into the waiting room in his usual blustery manner and had clearly not been briefed at how angry and upset I really was. He sat down and tried to placate me but I wasn't a girl who was for placating. I took a deep breath and explained the situation as I saw it. Quite simply, I was only proceeding with this round because he had given me the reassurance to do so, and part of that reassurance was tweaking the drugs to try to avoid previous complications. Now that was being called into question, or ignored.

Realising I was slightly agitated Prof went to speak to the team in the treatment rooms, to look through my file and learn more about what had happened. Returning he sat me down and advised me that having considered my file in great depth after speaking to us, he had over-ridden the audit meeting's recommendations and made the tweaks to the plan in an attempt to increase chances, although they were only tweaks. In preparing my drugs, the team had simply gone to the audit report and not noted the changes made in his letter and therefore there had been a clerical error, but that the recommendation was still as he had initially discussed with us. He acknowledged that they hadn't used the injections for some time but he thought that at the stage we were at, anything was worth trying and he still thought we should try them.

I felt more reassured. I was back on plan. It was designed around our journey and recommendations were being made for us after all, not just a textbook drugs course. There had been a mistake, an oversight and it was a good job I noticed, but for now, in front of kindly Prof and a nursing and admin team that I loved, all I cared about was that my anger had subsided, my mind was clearing and I was back on track with confidence. The drugs were changed and invoice corrected and after apologising to the team for my outburst and giving hugs all round, I calmly left the clinic feeling a great deal better about it all. I was thoroughly exhausted but in a far better place than I had been returning to the car just half an hour earlier.

By the time I got back to the office, my fury had returned. It was the thought that I nearly embarked on the cycle with the wrong drugs that incensed me. Whilst I knew that the slight tweak to the drugs might not have made any difference anyway, it was a huge part of my psychological state that got me into a frame of mind to risk embarking on the treatment at all. The drugs they suggested may have worked and certainly wouldn't have put me at any risk, but the thought that the tweaks made were done so from lessons learnt from our particular attempts in the past, gave us a huge positive boost. We may have found some element that may have let us down last time. The inconsistency made me furious and I paced up and down the boardroom in the office, crying as Emma listened to my insane ramblings. The thought came into my head once more that this would be the last time I could put myself and the team through this. It was all just too much and took too much out of me. It wasn't the plan, or the drugs; it was the impact on my mental state, my emotions and my sanity that was most troubling.

That night I started the injections. Holding the flesh I stuck the needle in without any trouble. It was almost like I was trying to hurt something else for not making me pregnant rather than my own body trying to get pregnant. Over the next few weeks, injection after injection, I tried not to get too caught up in the process each night and tried to make it seem like a matter of every day life. This was successful and the less I made out of doing them, the less they hurt and so the less I thought about them. They still hurt like hell, I still bruised badly and occasionally bled for a while but my reaction and attention paid to them was substantially less this time. It was just something I had to get on with.

I still felt flat, negative and whilst I never thought the treatment was a waste of time, for the first time I didn't feel one step closer to having a baby with every injection I put into myself. It was just something I had to do each night and so I did just that.

205

I carried on going to see Duncan at the gym but upped the effort and with every session I got more determined and more focussed. We put plenty of focus on my stomach and I was enjoying seeing the muscle look more and more defined each week. It was a great focus for me and it often felt that I could take my anger out on every chin lift I did. Through gritted teeth I'd be roaring and it felt good to let such noises out of my body. I felt in control during that hour and it felt good to have such a positive influence on my own body for a change.

During one session outside, when I was pushing myself doing some stretches and I wouldn't stop, I ended up having a heated debate with Duncan, about why I was pushing myself so hard of late. Duncan said: "You are blessed, you have Zac, this negativity is eating away at you, you need to be careful." I was incensed at his words. I knew I was blessed, I loved Zac more than anything in the world. I was so grateful to have him everyday. But this last year had made me so angry that I couldn't have what so many took for granted and the fact that I couldn't switch of that very desire drove me to distraction. I didn't want to feel this way, so angry, so sad, so helpless and useless. I didn't wake up each morning and decide to hate the world and concentrate on wanting other children instead of giving the one I had 100%. What's more, I certainly didn't want lecturing about it.

Once more I heard words escape my mouth that ordinarily I would have held back and swallowed: "It's alright for you saying that with three lovely kids and two beautiful grandchildren! I can't stop, I can't switch it off, I have to go on!" I was quick to apologise as soon as the words left my mouth. It was wrong for me to lash out and it was horrid of me to shout at Duncan especially, when he had done so much for me over the years and who I know only had my best interests at heart. I often wonder, but don't really want to know, what state I was in that evening for him to say what he did, but one thing for sure was that the treatment and failures were starting to eat into every part of my life and there wasn't much more I could take of it. I began to hate myself and how I was reacting. I hated the bitter feeling I was carrying that made me lash out at those who only wanted to help. But most of all I hated the feeling that I was someone who needed help. Was my life really that tragic?

Our fourth cycle

We cleared the diary and stayed close to home. It was November and nights were getting darker so it was easier to relax in at home together, but it was still hard to say no to nights out and get togethers with friends.

I hadn't really told many people we were doing the treatment again; such was the nonchalant attitude this time. In my mind, we were doing it again because we could and because we hadn't built ourselves up, so why not? It couldn't hurt. It might not work, but it wouldn't hurt us.

Eventually we ended up having to tell friends closest to us, as there were a few events and parties where it would have been suspicious or even rude if we didn't have a good excuse. One such occasion was Jason's friend's party. Jason went alone and said he felt difficult and awkward with me not there with him. We worried what his friends would think at my not making the effort, but in the end, we knew that we only entered into this again believing we were giving ourselves the best shot and if that meant I had to rest, then that was all that mattered. As it was, his friends were very understanding and despite being on his own for a change, Jason did have a great time.

Julie turned 40 that month and arranged a big couples night out in Leeds and we had to miss that too. Missing Jules' party was really disappointing and seeing the photographs of the antics that wild party girl got up to made it all the more disappointing, but once again, I was consoled by the fact that there would be more nights out in the future, but that we might never have another shot at IVF, so it had to be worth it.

By the weekend of Julie's night out, the drugs had really kicked in. I was feeling really sick and dizzy and could hardly eat which was most unlike me. I'm the only person I know who'd actually had perforated stomach ulcers and still didn't lose their appetite! So to be off my food was a real rarity and cause for concern.

I was on two lots of drugs, one set to boost the egg and follicle production and one lot to improve the quality of the eggs, which was one of the slight tweaks Prof had made. The nausea was unbaiting and it was with me from the moment I woke up. As the days went on it got stronger and stronger as did a massive headache that was almost debilitating.

That week, Zac was on his first half term holiday from school and I already felt emotional that I didn't have the holidays spare to be off with him as I needed the time off for after the transfer and couldn't afford any further days.

I had booked him into after school club for the week and took him there on the Monday morning. He had already started saying he hated the club, said it was too noisy and he had nobody to play with, so I was already apprehensive about him spending a whole week there, but wasn't about to let him see that. As it was though, my head was banging, I was on the verge of throwing my guts up and I had an early meeting in the office so I was hurriedly trying to settle him in. Despite rushing, I did notice that there was hardly any kids there and no boys his age to play with. I didn't have time or the strength to come up with an alternative solution so I just tried to soothe and settle him with one of the carers and assured him he'd have a great day. And yet it broke my heart. I could see he didn't want to go, had nobody to play with and as it was raining outside, would probably spend his day inside painting with the ladies. Hardly my budding football star's ideal day!

I got into the car and broke my heart. My poor baby. I felt terrible leaving him and felt even worse knowing that the reason I couldn't have the time off with him to do fun things was because I needed the time later for the transfer for the children I might not ever have. He couldn't have my time, but some unknown, unborn, chance of a second child could! Once again I was angry with myself for not giving my existing child my time. I was angry at my selfishness and guilty at my focussing in other directions away from him when he needed me. I called Jason and balled down the phone at him. I never offload my feelings like that but I was so upset I couldn't do anything else but cry down the phone at him. Little did I know his friend Jason was also in the car at the time. Whilst this was a little embarrassing it was also good fortune, as he told me about a holiday football club through Hull City that his boys had been on called Tigers Trust. Jason collected Zac as early as he could that afternoon and that evening we booked him onto Tigers Trust, from Wednesday to Friday.

On the Wednesday morning, Zac came to work with me for two hours until it was time to take him to the KC Stadium for the soccer school start at 10am. He sat by my desk colouring and amusing everyone, and as usual when he visited I was so proud of him and loved his funny little character. That morning however, I was feeling particularly poorly. I couldn't put my finger on it but as the morning progressed I just wanted to get Zac safely to the KC, so he was one less thing for me to think and worry about.

My head was banging so badly I could hardly see and I knew I was squinting. As we got into the car I suddenly felt really hot and didn't know whether I was going to faint, be sick or need to go to the toilet. Though we were only outside the office building I knew I didn't want to go back in whatever the outcome was going to be as we only had a single loo in the centre of the office, so I put my foot down and drove round the corner where there was fortuitously some public toilets. I grabbed Zac and ran to the toilets. I went to the toilet and without giving detail, lost a load that a bloke after a heavy night would be proud of. Where the hell did that come from? Zac was laughing his head off saying "God Mummy that stinks!" at the top of his voice! It was honestly horrendous. I was feeling faint and despite going to such an extent I didn't feel any better at all. We got back to the car but didn't get as far as the end of the street when I knew I was going to throw up. I grabbed at a carrier bag that was at Zac's feet. It had gym bra tops I was supposed to be taking back to the shop but I threw my guts up into it. I was sick three times in the car on the short drive to the KC and it was literally flying out of me. Both ends the effects were violent and had come from literally nowhere. It was horrific for me but must have been horrifying for my poor boy!

I was torn about what to do next and yet when I look at it now, in the cold light of day, it is obvious I should have just taken us both home. Zac would have eventually understood and he could have gone to Tigers Trust the next day. As it was, I was worried he would be upset as he'd been so looking forward to going, and I was also worried what they would think at work as I had appeared to be in good health when I left earlier just minutes earlier. I couldn't go back to the office with Zac because we were really busy and I wasn't in a fit state at that moment really to drive all the way home. I decided to try to get Zac to football and then I just had myself to sort out.

We parked next to the stadium by the Astroturf pitches and made our way towards a large gathering of 50 or 60 young boys and coaches. I had to pull Zac to one side immediately, as I threw up right next to the entrance. Then as I introduced Zac to the youngest group's coach, I had to step away and literally puke onto the edge of the Astroturf! It was a nightmare and I just wanted to try to get through the next few minutes, hand Zac over and get away as quickly as possible. The coach was so busy he didn't seem to notice that I'd thrown up and I felt so horrendous I didn't look around to see if anyone else had seen me. Then as I was filling in and signing the cheque in front of him, I threw up again, this time, as my stomach flipped and wretched I held the vomit in my mouth just long enough to do a ridiculous squiggle for my signature, and with just a few seconds to spare, I managed to turn, bend over and throw up again on the sidelines. With each wretch my head was banging and I just wanted to lie on the floor, which was by now apparently spinning beneath me.

I looked down into the big brown eyes of my little four year old and felt such shame and sorrow. I will never forget that day and how he looked at me. He seemed tiny and so young and to come to his first Tigers training session was such a big deal to him. The KC stadium was huge, the Astroturf pitches must have seemed vast and there were so many bigger, older boys I can only imagine it must have been terrifying.

The coach escorted all the younger boys along the Astroturf towards the indoor arena where they would be training for the day and as my little fella wandered off, with his boot bag and lunch box seemingly swamping his small frame, I could only chastise myself for not being there 100% for him. He needed reassuring, he needed to be confident and proud of his Mummy, he needed me and for weeks and months over the last year, I hadn't fully been there. I couldn't just leave him to march off into the unknown without making sure he felt all right being left there.

Today he needed me to be there for him, to hold his hand and reassure him. He was all on his own, without knowing a soul and all at the tender age of just four. He needed me sound of mind and strong in body, and today I was neither. I was hardly there for him at all. I dropped him off in a rush, whilst vomiting everywhere, with little capability of any reassurance or encouragement. Had he been older he would have undoubtedly been mortified by my behaviour! But he wasn't older, he was just four years old and he was still my baby boy.

Something changed that morning. It became clear that my priorities were all wrong. I was spending so long trying for another baby that I was neglecting the baby I had. For months I had been too sore and too tender to carry or hold him tightly and I missed that closeness and the comfort of his tiny body in my arms. I was undoubtedly missing instead of cherishing special moments as I had been so preoccupied for over 12 months now and I would never, ever get those moments back. And then here I was today, almost physically incapable of looking after him such was the impact those drugs were having on my body.

Enough was enough. He was my beautiful boy and he deserved the whole me, my complete focus. I started to realise that day that actually filling my life with Zac alone might not be such a bad thing. Perhaps I had always felt there was something missing because I had been focussing on something that wasn't there. Could it be that I could fill that void by giving my all to Zac and allowing him to complete my thoughts and fill my heart. I had felt that I had so much more love to give, but maybe if I stopped my quest and turned my full attention towards Zac, I would perhaps realise that there was so much more to him that I hadn't previously noticed and therefore so much more of him to love?

He was my baby. He meant the world to me and I wouldn't hesitate in saying I would do anything for him. But would I? Would I be able to give up trying for another child to be able to give him more?

What became clear that day, was that if we weren't successful this time, I wouldn't be jumping immediately into another attempt, if at all. It was having too big an impact on my family and my relationship with them. Sometime soon, if we continued as we had been doing, perhaps Zac would start to notice that I wasn't as active or connected as I had been and it would break my heart if he thought I was preoccupied with something else rather than him. I wouldn't want him to ever feel he wasn't enough, because he most certainly was everything to me. He had to be my priority. He had to be my main focus from here on in and if I thought for one moment that another round might have a negative impact on him, then my decision not to try again was made that day. Yes I wanted a sibling for him but I also wanted him to have a full time, full on Mummy. He deserved nothing less.

As ill as I felt, I watched his little figure tottering at the back of the long line of boys and I managed to walk behind the group following them to the arena, to make sure he was comfortable staying. He had said very little about me vomiting all over the place for the last half hour and I could only put that down to his nerves and focussing on what he was about to be doing himself.

As we got a little further down the path I could feel my stomach going again and I knew that having tried to keep the last two wretches down whilst talking to the coach, this time it was going to be a big one. I dashed into a small copse of trees next to the path, where I could just see the last few boys at the end of the line go past me, and there I threw my guts up. Thank God for those trees to hide in! What I didn't realise was that the path to the arena went past the copse and around the other side, so as I bent away from the back of the end of the line, I was now facing the front of the line with the two lead coaches looking at me in horror as I continued to vomit with great gusto.

I pulled myself together having finally finished vomiting and jogged as fast as I possibly could to rejoin the group at the back of the line, where one of the coaches was taking up the rear. I apologised and horrified at the thought that they may suspect I was drunk or hung over and that it therefore look badly on Zac for the rest of the week, I found myself explaining it away as morning sickness! I couldn't believe my own ears! And yet, the coaches seemed happy enough with the explanation and carried on as if nothing had happened.

Shaking and feeling delirious, I stood at on sidelines of the arena for ten minutes or so, as the boys got settled and started warming up. I told Zac I was going and as I was the only parent still there, he didn't seem bothered at all. I waved goodbye and made my way slowly back to the car, wondering how the hell we had survived the last half hour. My head was pounding and I was having trouble seeing very well by now. In fact I probably shouldn't have driven.

I parked the car outside the office and slowly made my way inside and into my office. Apparently I looked dreadful and after telling Emma that all I wanted to do was lie down, she grabbed my arm and suggested I do just that in the boardroom. She got her scarf to place under my head and I lay down with my coat on next to the radiator.

I was freezing cold, even my skin was cold and I couldn't stop aggressively shivering. I could hardly see and had become completely incoherent. I was completely empty so had finished vomiting thankfully but having been so sick I was now dizzy, completely drained and weak as a kitten. My arms and legs were aching and I just wanted to lay my head down, as it was so much effort just to hold it up. Emma was talking to me but I literally kept dozing off mid sentence.

Emma left me to sleep and told the team to leave me alone. They must have thought it bizarre that the boss was on the floor of the boardroom, hugging the radiator but if they did, nobody was saying so! What I didn't know was that Emma was so alarmed at my symptoms, she was hurriedly Googling the drugs that I was on and the severe side effects it described. She came back in to see me and suggested I call the clinic immediately as she was really worried. I could barely string a sentence together but she insisted I sit up and try to speak to them. I managed to dial the number and ask to be put through to Denise. I started trying to explain the state I was in and Denise very quickly advised me to stop taking the Metformin and to call them the next day to see how I was feeling. Emma took the phone and explained further the state I was currently in and thanked Denise for taking the call.

All I could do now was try to sleep; in fact I was incapable of anything else. Emma was asking what was happening with Zac and the small part of me that could still grasp a sense of reality and what was going on, broke a little bit more that afternoon as I realised I was simply unable to put my thoughts together sufficiently to come up with a plan of how to collect him. I could remember where he was, and I eventually told them a time but as for any other arrangement I was incapable of making a plan to collect and care for him. I cried and know that had I been in any more of a lucid state I would have cried some more. I wasn't in a fit state to sort out care for my child! I had to rely on my colleagues to go and collect him, call his dad and make arrangements to get us both picked up from the office. I would have been mortified at the time had I been feeling any better, but as time went on and days went by, the full realisation as to the full extent of the impact that the drugs were having on us all, began to terrify me.

I spent the whole afternoon on the floor in the office. Emma and Anna went to collect Zac and then the team amused him in the office until Jason was able to collect us both at the end of the day. I stumbled out of the door with the assistance of Jason as I could still hardly see and was feeling extremely dizzy.

That was undoubtedly the worst day during the entire IVF process and one I will never forget. It changed my view on whether we should keep trying for a baby. I understood more fully other people's experience of my journey better from their perspective, particular Emma and Dom's. But most importantly it reignited that fiercely protective maternal instinct I had for Zac, my child, that I had feared had started to wane and wasn't needed as he grew up and became more independent. He did still need me and I did still need to be there for him.

Final stages of our final attempt

As soon as I stopped the Metformin I quickly felt a lot better. I couldn't believe how poorly it had made me and on describing my symptoms to Denise a couple of days later, she determined that I was obviously really sensitive to drugs and had clearly had an extreme reaction. As she said, the addition of the Metformin was merely a small tweak to the plan in an attempt to improve the quality of the eggs and stopping the drug now wouldn't impact the cycle in any way. It was far better to stop the drug and risk a lower quality of egg rather than keep going with it making me as poorly as it was. There was no decision to make and it was clear I couldn't take it any more. However, I was totally fine with the decision when the next scan showed that my follicles were growing nicely and slowing down the drugs was obviously working. So, I carried on with the injections and we started to plot the dates for the egg retrieval and transfer.

The dates on the fourth cycle seemed to come round quicker than they had done in previous attempts. Perhaps it was because I was less anxious and not as focussed on what we were doing, but before we knew it I was wrapping up projects at work, doing handovers to the new team members before my week long holiday and preparing to go to the clinic in the morning for retrieval.

Jason and I were both quiet that morning. We had discussed the effects of the drugs at length a few times and we had both felt that the treatment was taking its toll on both of us. By now it was November and as the first transfer had been November the previous year, that meant we had had four attempts in just 13 months! That was some going by anyone's book! It didn't ever feel like it was such a mission doing it so many times in such a short space of time, in fact at the time, I wouldn't have dreamt of not having another go straight after I had failed on the previous attempt. Yet that morning, looking back at the journey across the previous year, we both knew that we were nearing the end of this journey and it made us slightly anxious at the prospect of not visiting the clinic again, and all that then being in that situation might entail for us. We wanted another child for our family but we also wanted the family that we had to be happy.

Prof came to greet us in the waiting room and welcomed us to the clinic. He was on countdown to his retirement and during the previous months had often amused me with his instant knowledge of precisely how many days he had left until he retired. That morning he greeted us with the usual announcement of the number of days and I remember distinctly saying to him as we walked through the double doors towards the treatment rooms "This better work this time Prof, because if not, you're not going anywhere, you won't be retiring!"

I was sore as always following the retrieval but it had been a success and Denise was able to collect 22 eggs, 14 of which we were subsequently told had successfully fertilised to a quality standard. As ever, I was extremely lucky to have so many good quality eggs, very lucky indeed.

Five days later, we received the call from the embryologist and once more we took the call, anxious to hear that we had at least one to transfer. After such a traumatic and painful build up this time, I couldn't bear it if we should fall at this final hurdle and not have any embryos to transfer.

We had two. We had two excellent blastocyst embryos! For the first time through this whole fourth attempt I was giddy. Jason and I had dared to discuss what we would do if there was more than one embryo and had already agreed that if we had more than enough to freeze we would do that and if we had two we would insist on having both put back. I was firm down the phone when I said to the embryologist that we wanted both putting back. I could hear myself telling her this was our last shot, our final attempt and I didn't want to be hijacked in theatre to discuss it, I definitely wanted two putting back in. I asked her to please explain to Denise that I didn't want to discuss it when I arrived as we had already thought long and hard about it. This was our last go and we really wanted the very best chance.

Jason and I hugged for what seemed like the longest time. Was that out of excitement or fear or both? We were both terrified of the outcome this time and as much as we had made little fuss about the treatment so far, today was what it was all about and the enormity wasn't lost on us. As much as my numbness had smothered my sadness, it had by no means dampened

215

my longing and here, stood with just hours until the final stages of what was increasingly feeling like our final attempt to have another child, I ached and longed for that child more than I had ever done before.

When we arrived and were escorted to our bay in the treatment room by the ever-lovely team, we were both nervous and excited. Denise popped her head round the curtain and said she knew we wanted both embryos put back, that it was fine to do so and we wouldn't be discussing it any further. I found myself trying to justify to her why we insisted on two and also why I had made a point of insisting we shouldn't discuss it in theatre when I was on the phone. I didn't want Denise to feel bullied or that I didn't acknowledge or appreciate her opinion and advice. Quite the contrary. She had been my rock throughout all the treatment and I valued her more than anyone on the team, perhaps more than Prof in some ways. She was confident, assured; straight talking and I trusted her implicitly. As it was, she didn't seem to mind our decision or how she heard about it and as ever, she went about her business readying the team for theatre with great efficiency and nothing more was said.

One, then two were successfully and relatively easily transferred in. "Hello you two!" I whispered. I had so wanted to take my mobile in to take photographs of them on the screen in their embryo stage, as I had been too nervous to do so in previous attempts. As it was, I was again too nervous to ask if this was OK and weirdly as I sat in recovery, contemplating the last hour and trying to decipher if I was actually excited or nervous, suddenly that photograph wasn't important.

I wanted a child. That feeling had never left me and I had gone to hell and back during the last year to try to fulfil that desire. If we weren't successful this time, a photograph of yet another two unsuccessful embryos would only serve as a painful reminder and if we were to be successful, I would hopefully have new images created every day before my very eyes that I could enjoy, instead of that photograph.

Could we ever imagine a positive result?

Jason took me home and once more I took up my place on the sofa, wrapped myself in the blanket and rested for the weekend. This time I rested better than I had previously. I didn't go anywhere and didn't do anything. We had put everything into this last round and there was nothing more important or that couldn't wait.

One of Jason's longest standing friends was getting married in Leeds the weekend after transfer and a few weeks before, once we'd had confirmation of our treatment dates, we had let them know that I wouldn't be able to make it. I was gutted to miss their celebration but there was no way I was going anywhere during that week. I urged Jason to attend on his own as afterall it was his friend and I thought the time away with the lads would do him the world of good. He had a great time, caught up with old friends but said it all felt very strange without me by his side. Then talking to a wife of another of his friends, she told him she was pregnant with their second. Of course he was thrilled and hugged them both as he gave his congratulations. Yet as he told me all about it when he arrived home later, I could see in his face the blow this had been on hearing that news that night. He was trying to have one night away, one night off from all of this and the reminder of what was going on at home thumped him straight in the gut as he held himself up at the bar. There was no escape. There is never any escaping it.

As this plan included the highest dose of HCG possible in the injection rather than pessary format, we had been told that rather than find out the result through a pregnancy test in two weeks, we could only find out via a blood test and scan in nine weeks time! Nine weeks! It seemed like a lifetime away but weirdly it was also less pressure and less frustrating than the usual two week wait. It was ages off so it was easier to forget about it and after the initial weekend of relaxing, I got back to my usual business and activities, albeit perhaps in a slower, less stressful way.

Days passed and weeks started to pass and eventually after five weeks I was due at the clinic for a blood test. I went and had bloods taken on Wednesday and again on Friday morning. Denise was clear to reiterate that this was merely to check my hormone levels and as they would show high for HCG anyway, it would be impossible to say if I was pregnant. What they could perhaps indicate was however, whether I wasn't pregnant.

That Friday seemed to drag, slow second by slow second. Was this the day when it was all going to end? To stop. To finish and be all over once and for all? I had a client meeting close to home at lunchtime and had been advised to call the clinic at 3pm for the result. The meeting was with a client I enjoyed working for and someone I really got on with so it was easy to enjoy my time and to take my mind off the impending news we were about to hear, but as the afternoon wore on, I could feel myself getting increasingly agitated and nervous about coming home. As could probably be predicted, I was late and was racing home to get back for 3pm. I called Jason and he was already at home and inevitably scolding me for not leaving sooner. I deserved it, I should have made my excuses and left but it wasn't that easy to end the meeting and I certainly couldn't have given the real reason as an excuse.

I will always remember driving down a particular road near our house that has expanse of open fields to either side, the beautiful rolling hills of the Yorkshire Wolds ahead of you and the effect of a roller coaster as the tarmac rises and falls away as you head a mile or two towards the next junction. I remember getting more and more nervous as I was just two minutes from home. Two minutes from finding out whether our journey had ended.

"Please God, I'm not asking you for a baby anymore. I'm not asking you for a positive result today. I won't waste my prayers asking for a baby any more. If I'm not meant to be blessed with another baby, please, please send your blessings and take the longing away. Please God, I'm begging you, let it all be over and take it away today. Let it be the end. If I'm not meant to have another baby today then please stop me from wanting one, that's all I ask. Amen."

I will never forget that journey, that road or those words. I meant it. I had literally had enough and wanted my life back. My lovely full life with Jason and Zac. I couldn't do it any more and I wanted the longing to go away.

The end of the road

It was just gone three and we called Denise. I could hardly breathe let alone speak. We were both stood next to the island in the kitchen; with me talking into the phone but holding it close enough so Jason could hear. Denise explained that they had my second lot of blood test results back to compare with Wednesday's results and they had increased in levels, which was a very positive sign. So it wasn't a definite negative. I held my breath as she went on. Whilst they obviously couldn't confirm that we were pregnant, which we knew, the reading was exceptionally high for this early on, which she said could indicate positive results.

Jason and I looked at each other and we both knew the other one had no idea what was being said to us. Denise went on to explain that whilst it was good news that the result had gone up, the amount by which it had actually increased was such that she recommended a scan, which would be the only way to confirm a positive result. A scan? Really? But we have four more weeks to wait? I could hardly believe my ears. This was insane! I quickly asked when and was floored when she replied that the clinic was closed but she was still there working and was prepared to stay there to scan us that afternoon if we could get there!

Our lives had just fast-forwarded one month in a split second and we were both completely in shock. Of course we would come and we would come straight away! How lovely was that of Denise to offer to do that for us? I was overwhelmed by her kindness and consideration for our feelings that afternoon and in my shock at being offered the scan I had completely forgotten about Zac and the school run at 3.30pm. It was Friday after all and my day for pick up!

I called our neighbour Sara, explained the situation and asked if she would mind collecting Zac and looking after him for a short time whilst we went to the clinic. Having then thought some more about it, Zac hadn't been collected by anyone else before and was never very comfortable when plans changed at the last minute, so Jason and I decided to go to the school, meet him at his classroom then explain that we had an appointment and take him to Sara to bring him home.

He was delighted to see us both waiting for him and came bounding over excited that we would be going home together. It came as somewhat of a blow to him therefore when we told him he was going home with Sara and he cried his eyes out in the back of her car as we waved goodbye. We thought we were doing the right thing in meeting him and yet, still we had managed to upset him. I couldn't talk to Sara about what we were doing and fortunately she didn't ask. She just hugged me and wished us luck. As Jason and I hurried back to our car in the car park, I was trying to hold back the tears that were now beginning to surface as I recalled my little boy crying. I was a nervous wreck, my hands were shaking and I was wringing my fingers round and round.

We didn't know what to expect or what we were to be told but it felt like the most nervous and excited mix of emotions I had ever felt in my life. My heart was pounding so hard in my chest it almost hurt. Denise had given us the private phone number of the office to call when we arrived as the reception was closed and she warmly welcomed us into the clinic.

In the sonographer's room that I was so familiar with, I climbed on the bed and Denise readied the equipment, turning the screen towards her. It was uncomfortable as usual but I was solely focussed on Denise's face. Jason squeezed my hand and he too focussed on Denise's face.

"One, two, hhmmm it looks like there may be three sacks in there."

"What?" I exclaimed!

Denise looked again and after some consideration said: "Well there are definitely signs of a pregnancy and I would guess that there is two there, although there may be three. If I was to guess at this early stage I would say you have two."

We were pregnant. We had been scanned and it was true, we were actually pregnant. We didn't know whether to celebrate yet but initially it was all I could do to muster an intake of breath. We were elated but as reminded by

Denise, we knew we had a long way to go and as with every stage of every round of IVF, any positive news is quickly quashed with a blanket, as you know you have to face the next hurdle. So we were pregnant today and there might be three babies or none of those may end up being viable. Three or none. It was a spectrum that was too broad to contemplate, to take in, and to understand. We held each other and hugged as we made our way slowly back down the now familiar corridor towards the exit. We had hugged and thanked Denise for her time and her kindness and said we would make an appointment to revisit for a confirmation scan in 10 days time.

As I went across the road to collect Zac later that evening, my head was spinning with the news we had heard and yet my priority now was to get to my son and give him a big hug and check he was OK. Of course he was fine, in fact he was having a great time and wouldn't come downstairs to go home. I stood in Sara's kitchen feeling like I had been punched in the face and I couldn't help but share my surreal news. So there are signs of three but then none of them might be viable. Well that was how we saw it. We could end up being Swiss Family Robinson or it could just still be the three of us forever more. I could feel my eyes welling up but I couldn't determine if it was joy, excitement or fear.

They were the longest 10 days of my entire life. Our minds would wander from one potential scenario to the other and the contrast between them was almost too much to consider. All I kept thinking was if there were three, how the hell do you ever leave the house and do anything? And yet, such worries might be wasted, as there was still a real possibility that this early into a pregnancy, none of the three might survive.

Ten days later and we were to find out. The words "There's one and..... there's another one." will stay with me all my days. After checking everywhere for a third, the sonographer finally confirmed that we were having twins and she could see two heartbeats. We were seven weeks pregnant with twins who both had strong, healthy heartbeats!

We left the scanning room and outside met Debbie, Dawn and Caroline who could see it was a positive result from our faces and each warmly embraced us as they congratulated us both. Dawn took us into one of the meeting rooms, where she gave us paperwork to give to our GP and once again gushed with her excitement at our news.

We walked out into the reception and through tears I held up two fingers in the Victory V sign at Roxanne, Karen and Caroline in the office and mouthed "there's two!" They too came out to warmly embrace us and congratulate us. It had been a long, eventful journey and they had been with us all the way. It was lovely to celebrate with them and finally to share some good news.

We walked out of the door and as it closed behind us Jason took me in his arms and we both wept. I cried my eyes out and thought I might lose my legs I felt that overcome by the news. We held each other for the longest time and then, still embracing each other with both arms, walked slowly towards the exit. We were leaving the clinic for the last time, with two heartbeats, two smiles and one fantastic big brother waiting for us at home.

Epilogue

On the 12th May 2013, Anya Elizabeth Rose and Xavier Andrew were born into our lives. At just 29 weeks I went into early labour and both babies were delivered within two hours by emergency caesarean section just six minutes apart. Anya weighed 2lb 7oz and Xavier weighed 2lb 12oz. They spent the next 10 weeks two floors up from the IVF clinic in the Neo-natal Intensive Care Unit at Hull Royal and eventually, we left through the same main doors, passing the IVF clinic on the left, to come home on the 19th July. We were complete.

Reflections

If the truth is to be told, I always struggled with how I might end this story. When I was writing it, I didn't know the actual ending myself as I started writing just as I was about to commence my first IVF cycle. I didn't know if we would be successful or if it would all end with just the three of us. What I did know for sure was that I didn't ever want it to be a story with a 'happily ever after' ending. One where a baby popped out, we were happy and dreams always come true, the end. I was always nervous about the ending, not least because I wanted to know how my story would go, but I also was adamant that I never wanted to ostracise anyone who didn't have a happy ending, whose fairy tale didn't come true. I wanted to give an honest account of Secondary Infertility for everyone who was struggling, and for some, unfortunately the end of the story isn't always a baby.

It was only as I was drawing to a close, a few months after the babies' arrival, that a close friend insisted I had to say we had been successful and to tell people we had our babies. That was the truthful ending after all. People want to know and people need hope she said! I agreed but I only wrote a short paragraph as I felt the birth and subsequent story was a whole different journey and not one I felt relevant to the readers of this particular book. It was only sometime later that two other friends suggested I write a chapter reflecting back on the journey, giving more information about what happened next and offering my thoughts on what I learned and how it affected us.

Each night I say to all three children: "Night night, I love you, my dreams come true." I say it because I mean it, they are. They are my absolute dreams come true and prayers answered. Yet I know I'm fortunate and in giving the insight in this chapter, I in no way want to paint a perfect ending that might give an unrealistic glossy finish to fertility tales, but I do hope it offers hope, strength and faith to anyone who has found our story meaningful.

What happened next?

The pregnancy was fairly straightforward, though of course with twins everybody was extra cautious and I quickly grew to quite a size! In fact I was as big at 29 weeks with them as I was at 37 weeks when Zac was born.

Jason and I struggled for a long time to get our heads round the fact that we were actually pregnant. It was often too much to grasp that we were really going to have one other child, let alone two!

As soon as we had the seven-week scan, we were excited to tell our closest friends and families, confirming that there were two viable pregnancies with two strong heartbeats. After everything we had been through, we didn't want to wait, didn't see the point in keeping everyone guessing, when to be quite honest, the look of shock on our faces gave it away.

We were both excited but cautious to tell Zac. It was still early days, there was so much that could go wrong and neither of us wanted to put him through any pain that he didn't need to experience just yet. At the same time, he was astute and sometimes nosey and I was adamant that we should be the ones to tell him and explain what was happening, rather than him overhear a conversation or for somebody else to let it slip.

Both grinning, we sat him down, and put his hand on my tummy. "Inside Mummy's tummy there's two babies!" Quizzically he said: "We're going to have not just one, but two babies?" He couldn't get his head round two, we'd only ever discussed one with him really, so he couldn't understand how on earth two got in there! He was pleased but confused and not sure what it all meant really, but it was delightful to watch his little face light up and his smile grow as he tried to work it all out. We later found out he ran up to tell his teacher first thing the next day and told her all about it with great excitement.

We told wider family and friends on Christmas Day, ringing them all with our amazing news, which was made all the better for our family members, as my brother Andrew and Kate also announced that they too were expecting another baby, just 8 weeks later. Boy were we all lucky that we had been successful this time, perhaps most of all my brother, who had been dreading telling us their great news for days, in case we weren't pregnant!

We visited my cousin Paula over Christmas and she brought out the double buggy she used for Zoe and Elin for me to try. I freaked! It was all too surreal. Holding the handles, looking down at the two empty spaces and listening to Paula's giddy descriptions of how you folded it seemed all too much. It was like standing in someone else's shoes and living someone else's life. Paula then freaked Jason out by putting Elin's new babies in his arms – triplets! They were lifelike tiny newborns, way too realistic for Jason and I to cope with and as he sat holding all three and then just two of them, Jason's face was an absolute picture. One of acute embarrassment tinged with fear! It was as terrifying as it was funny.

Whilst I grew, so did our anxiety. I was excited but nervous. We weren't sure whether to find out the genders at the 20 week scan but one day in Mothercare, I noticed two tiny vests, one with pink hearts and one with blue stars. I realised that I really did need to start believing because we had an awful lot of preparation to do. We were unable to really plan because we couldn't get our heads round it and dare not believe it would happen. Not knowing the combination, whether, two boys, two girls or one of each just added to the mystery and 'unreal' situation. We truly didn't mind what the combination was, we just needed to know, to believe.

As the sonographer scanned round my belly, I spotted that the first was a boy straight away, and now having met Xavi, it's true that he is definitely a show off. It took a little longer to see the second as they were a little more shy but when we both heard the words "yes, I'm pretty certain, yes, it's a girl!", Jason and I both cried. It sounds daft to write that it was a fairytale ending, but a boy and a girl seemed like the perfect combination for us. We would have loved both boys, yet two girls together would have been super special too, but our combo of a boy to play with Zac and a girl to shop with Mummy seemed so perfect we could hardly believe our luck. A baby boy AND a baby girl. Our joy was overwhelming.

Jason drove me straight back to Mothercare where I bought the two tiny vests, one pink hearts and one blue stars and I bought two tiny hats to match too. Placing both hats on my now large tummy, I walked into the office and shared the news. I sent a photo of the hats on my tummy to friends and family with the caption: "look what we just found out!" It was surreal.

We started to narrow down our name selection which again, helped us to take in and believe what was soon about to happen. Then we thought we should start seriously looking at buying equipment, changing the car for one that had space for three seats in the back, and preparing the nursery for two cribs!

By the beginning of May, I was starting to struggle a little with the weight of the babies. They weren't huge and neither was my bump compared to some twin pregnancies and I was still only 28 weeks but the pressure on my pelvis was sometimes unbearable. Our little boy was at the top kicking hell out of my ribs and our little girl was down at the bottom pressing on my pelvis and cervix, so much so that by now, I was having to wear a supportive pelvic girdle. It was the least attractive but the most magnificent contraption ever! The pain had been so great one day that I literally couldn't put a foot to the floor and had to crawl from the kitchen back to my desk on my hands and knees!

Apart from the pelvic pain and tightness across my abdomen as it stretched, I felt great and the babies were nice and lively. I did start to wonder if I would ever actually reach July though. The babies 40-week due date was 31st July but that seemed an eternity away and I literally thought I'd pop well before even the first of July the way I was going. I kept saying to people "I'm not sure I'm going to make July!"

I had a routine scan one Thursday, which went well, but confirmed Placenta Preavia. My obstetrician, who thankfully I knew from the IVF clinic, wasn't worried but advised that he would book me in for a C-section at 38 weeks, which would have been 18th July. It was exciting to start to focus on the birth, the arrival of our much longed for babies, but it was also great to hear that they were doing well and cooking nicely.

Four days later, Sunday 12th May, I was curled up under a blanket snuggling with Zac on the sofa, watching the 'Got To Dance' final we had recorded on TV, when I instantly knew that the warm 'whoooosh' feeling was my waters breaking. I calmly got up and walked quickly to the toilet where, before I could sit down, another whoooosh came, but this time splattered the floor and walls with more water and what seemed like pints of fresh blood. I closed the door so Zac couldn't see and shouted for Jason to call 999. I wasn't going to make June never mind July! The twins were on their way.

Two hours later, after a blue light dash to Hull Royal, we were in theatre, nervously waiting to meet our babies. We were 29 weeks to the day.

Zac was being cared for across the road at Sara's and Jason rang Jo to ask her to drive my Mum across, which she did and they then both stayed and looked after Zac for the next few days.

I'll never forget Anya's little kitten cry as she came out first, it was the most beautiful and welcome sound I have ever heard. Xavi was stuck and took some wriggling to get out but just 6 minutes later, we welcomed our second son. There was no sound and we later learned that he had to be worked on as they intrabated his tiny 2lb body. The next few hours are a blur for me. The neo-natal team were on hand to take over and they whisked our precious babies off to the Neo-natal Intensive Care Unit, stopping the transport incubators briefly by my head for me to see the tiny knitted bonnets peeping out.

The Hull NICU team cared for our babies and our family for the next ten weeks and on July 25th, just one week before their actual due date, we eventually took our babies home. During those weeks, Zac proudly told everyone about his new brother and sister and his Reception teachers and classmates made beautiful cards that were up in my hospital room, then in our lounge. Some days he was indifferent and frustrated and just wanted it to be the three of us again, wanting Mummy to himself. Other days he didn't want to leave the unit, preferring to stay with me, helping me and busying himself with little jobs for the babies. The NICU team were as wonderful with him as they were with the little ones, drawing with him, teaching him how to wash his hands like a doctor and involving him fully so that he never ever felt left out.

Jason had quickly texted Dom and Emma to tell them I wouldn't be coming in, understatement of the year! They both came to visit on the first Thursday and Dom had printed out a photo I had sent them of each baby and put them in a frame, with another frame in which he'd printed and mounted their names. I cried, as he said I would, but it was a lovely affirmation that we did actually have our babies, it had happened and they were real. I still have those frames and will never forget what they meant, and what he did for me that day.

There were scary times, touch and go moments, endless examinations that tested Jason and I to the limit. It was hard going for sure, but we also had some wonderful memories of our NICU journey, met new life long friends and it taught us so much about the value of the NHS and the wonderful people who looked after us.

For the second time, our lives were touched by a team that helped fulfil our dreams, this time to save rather than create our family, and once again we were overwhelmingly indebted. As the babies' graduation day drew closer, I became extremely anxious that I needed each and every member of the team to know how much I loved them and how thankful I was. A box of chocolates somehow didn't seem to do the job! That first year, with the help of family and friends, we raised £52,722 for the NICU team to buy a new transport incubator, cooling mat and a cooling cap to try to express our gratitude. One of the nurses reassured me that every NICU nurse understands how grateful we are because if they didn't, they couldn't do their job. I was pleased to hear her confirm that, but we wanted each and every member of that team that will touch that equipment to know that it was donated to the unit in their name, for what they all do each day and that they are hugely appreciated.

Three years on

And so, as the babies are now three, Zac is now nine and we are six and a half years on from when our journey for a second child started, it's interesting to read back on what happened, read each chapter as if it were yesterday yet also strangely feels like it was a different lifetime.

Now, it's like we were always going to have three children, that Zac was always going to have siblings to love and annoy him and yet, the truth behind everyday life still doesn't escape either Jason or I.

It is inconceivable to imagine our lives as anything other than a family of five. Jason and I, with our three children. Three children!? I still sometimes look at them all, especially the twins, and ask myself "how did that happen?" Our house is busy, noisy and, those who know us well would say crazy. It really is hard to ever remember when people didn't think of us that way.

But there was a long time when we never thought it would happen, when we began to imagine life fast forward as just the three of us, of Zac growing up with just Jason and I. Whilst we enjoy life thoroughly now, it's important to remember where we were, where we all came from and I have promised myself that all three children will always know what we went through. I want them to know how much they were wanted, how much we loved them before we knew them but most of all to know about the struggles some people still go through everyday just to have a family and that others are sadly unable to. I particularly want them to know what they inspired in Jason and I and how their very existence has driven us in a new direction.

Writing our story was certainly therapy for me, just as the fundraising was therapy following our NICU experience. I started writing as we embarked on our first round of IVF so it's strange to read now some of the more prophetic paragraphs, now we know the outcome.

Zac asking for not just one baby but a brother and a sister, and the brother better be good at football! That's exactly what he got! Me feeling that I was always going to have twins and Emma saying to me during the second cycle that she thought I'd have twins – and I did! There were times when we conceded that it might never happen and yet to read some of these paragraphs, it's seems bizarre now knowing that it did!

After finishing the book, I was overwhelmingly driven to get it published to try to share the story and help others who might be struggling to extend their family. (It had also been a lifelong bucket list entry for me to have a manuscript published). Each night as I sat with the laptop, tapping away till the early hours, I imagined a couple cuddling together on a sofa, feeling lonely and guilty for wanting another child, and with each word I typed I wanted to reach out and tell them, they should not feel guilty, they were not alone and it was OK to want more.

I launched a website and Facebook page and immediately that evening, I was overwhelmed with the positive response. I knew I had done a great thing by sharing my story, it was job done. Or rather as it turned out, the first job done. The positive feedback only gave me more to do!

Years before, sitting for literally hundreds of hours pouring my heart out into that laptop, it often felt like the loneliest place on the planet. I will never forget the moment I read a paragraph in Zita West's Guide to IVF (bible) that mentioned existing parents often had a feeling of guilt. At last somebody understood. That was me! I was shocked as I read the words but I was also immensely comforted. I'll also remember the shock at learning that our situation actually had a name 'Secondary Infertility'. At the time I felt relief as at last I felt 'defined', part of a group and suddenly not so alone. And now I had been able to do that for someone else.

In the first six hours of that first evening of the website launch on Facebook, it already had 50 likes, 14 shares and I had 4 orders for my book! And yet it was the 3 comments made on the homepage that meant the most.

To receive feedback that day from 3 people who were at the time in a similar situation and to have them overwhelmingly thank me for sharing my story is one of the strangest and most rewarding feelings I have ever felt. In the words of one:

"I honestly can't relate to that enough. You have captured how I'm sure a million women feel. At a daunting yet exciting time, this had given me so much positivity for the future. I said to my husband tonight that it's so liberating to feel like 'Yes! Someone finally gets how I feel!' I still have hope and it's been made stronger today by your words. I honestly feel like the universe arranged for you to press that button today just as I needed it. Today you have become my absolute hero. Honestly what you've done for me just today has been a total gift."

I had always dreamed of getting this book published but that night, those words meant more to me than any Amazon listing or book in my hand. My dream of talking to that couple on a sofa somewhere and getting them to finally feel that they weren't alone, was achieved that first night. I knew how she felt and she now felt understood. She didn't feel so alone anymore and I hoped she could start to shake off a little of the guilt she had been carrying round.

Yet I felt immensely sad that despite launching on the World Wide Web, that girl lived just 10 minutes away and I'd known here for 14 years. We lived so near, yet when you are struggling alone, we live so far away. And so the dream and ambition grew just as soon as the first dream had been achieved. I needed to reach more couples.

When the sixth publisher knock back came, their words didn't put me off, they ignited a further fire in me that continues to burn and propelled my life in a whole new direction I could never have dreamed possible. They told me they loved so much about the book, that I would be great in helping to market it but that I had failed two of their essential tick boxes in the final editorial commissioning meeting.

They didn't feel there was enough of a market as "nobody searched for Secondary Infertility on Amazon and the last Secondary Infertility memoir only sold 26 copies in 10 years!". I was livid.

I spent £20,000, underwent 4 rounds of IVF and wrote this book before ever stumbling across the term 'Secondary Infertility' so of course never searched Amazon using it, nor Google for that matter! I searched for 'Trying for another baby', 'Wanting a second child'. If I had known the term, I may have found some information that would have hugely helped, but then again I may not have felt compelled to write our story had I realised I wasn't the only one in this situation. But the fact I didn't know the term, the fact that I felt so alone and so horribly guilty and the additional fact that after launching a website about my book I was inundated with girls thanking me as they too were feeling alone, only fuelled my drive to get the book published.

I've learned so much since finishing the book and feel a real sense of purpose and responsibility to raise the profile of Secondary Infertility. This was my story but is seemed to be that the story of Secondary Infertility was far greater and more important.

Secondary Infertility is still infertility. In many ways the symptoms and journey are much the same as those struggling to conceive a first child. Investigations, treatments and disappointment are common in both Primary and Secondary Infertility. You are still struggling to make a baby. It's pain, just a different pain.

It is difficult enough to admit that your body is letting you down. It's often excruciating to share your pain at yet another failed cycle and it's harder than anyone realises listening to friends and family announcing a surprise pregnancy. When you already have a family but would like another child, there is a level of understanding that is absent. You have a child, so you should be happy that at least you have one, or that's how others see it. Sometimes having and loving that first child is the biggest driver for wanting another, in that you want to provide a sibling.

There isn't a quota on having babies. Just because you have one doesn't mean you shouldn't want or have another. Just as your wanting another won't prevent someone else from conceiving their first child. Yet you feel greedy for admitting you want more. You have every right to have another child and you have every right to expect some sympathy and support when Mother Nature isn't playing ball. Afterall, it's the same old Mother Nature in all of us that kick starts the hormones and rattles our ovaries, teasing us with the desire for children in the first place!

Secondary Infertility has become a taboo, a shameful condition, one that sufferers feel guilty about having or talking about because they are the first to realise how lucky they are. They don't need to be told to focus on the child they know they are already blessed with.

Anyone struggling to conceive another child, doesn't want to offend Primary Infertility sufferers, indeed many struggled the first time themselves, as we had. Too often they are couples who choose to pretend they aren't trying so as not to offend or to avoid confrontation. They struggle in silence. They feel alone. They in turn reinforce the stigma from which they feel so much pressure.

1 in 6 couples struggle with Infertility and 1 in 3 couples undergoing fertility treatment are struggling with Secondary Infertility* and probably feel alone. But that statistic itself is a contradiction. 1 in 3 are obviously not alone! That figure cannot be ignored, it's far too many people.

Today, I still see it as my mission to help bring greater understanding, far greater empathy and much wider knowledge of the term Secondary Infertility and all its complexities. We need to help bring the subject and it's sufferers out of the dark and into a society where it's OK to say "I want another child."

I am writing a second book, a self-help guide to Secondary Infertility, I have a website and manage social media pages, I write for Fertility Road magazine, I support the Hull IVF unit as a Patient Representative and work closely with Fertility Network UK as Media Volunteer on the subject. I also speak to IVF students and drug companies to give an insight into what fertility treatment is like from a patient's perspective, and as the story is spreading, the media interview requests are increasing. These opportunities are priceless to me and I talk to whoever will listen to try to raise the profile of those two little words, Secondary Infertility, as much as possible.

---

* Source: fertilityIQ.com

What did I learn?

Every baby changes your life, but without doubt, all three of our children and the fight to have them, changed and shaped my life. I view the world and those around me completely differently. I view my own life, purpose and value completely differently too. If I had had three Bacardi Breezers, conceived naturally three times and popped out my three babies with one push year after year, I would be a completely different person to the one I am today.

Would I change it? Sometimes yes to be truthful. Not the outcome of course, but the journey, in some ways yes. I love what we have, our values, our beliefs, the insight into worlds we never knew existed definitely, but there are of course times when I still wish we had twenty grand in the bank or wonder what I used to fill my brain or life with before we went through all of this. Would ignorance be bliss? When I read back and remember some of the darker days, yes sure, being brutally honest, I do wish we hadn't had to go through them, wish I was less lined and more pert! I'd change some parts if I could for sure, and that's just the honest truth.

And yet, every step, every painful event was just a chapter or step in life. And this was my destiny. I consider myself very, very fortunate. I don't write about our experience for sympathy, far from it. I am very blessed and certainly don't need sympathy. I write because there are those still battling and there are those who have had to give up the battle. Some can't tell their story, either too pained or simply too shy. I can, and I will, in the hope that more understanding is given to this common situation.

It really is OK to want another child. It's a natural urge, it's not greedy, not selfish, it's a human instinct that you can't fight.

I also want to break the taboos of 'fertility'. Just because you might need intervention, it doesn't mean you deserve another child any less or that you or that child has any less value. "Are they IVF?" is sometimes said in such an insulting, demeaning way, almost referring to a child as a fake, or an easy shortcut, especially when you have twins. How lovely if fertility treatment could be embraced and celebrated, rather than the negative always being the focus.

I've also thought long and hard since reading back the pages just before our fourth cycle. We really did say that was our last attempt and I remember really meaning it too. We had given it everything in those 13 months and felt spent in every sense. I always say now that had we not been successful who knows, we may well have had another go, but at that time, I really did believe I couldn't continue any longer.

I specifically remember re-evaluating my feelings. I was well into writing this book at the time and it already had the working title 'More Love To Give' as I felt this perfectly summed up how I felt at the time. Yet I do distinctly remember, after the incident at Zac's football training and then in the office, considering that perhaps, when I felt I had more love to give, I was sometimes not looking in the right places to focus that love. That actually, I had spent so long chasing another baby, I could in fact be denying Zac more love and attention he needed or deserved. Sometimes wanting something so badly can turn your head away from what you have already. It truly felt that this was happening towards the end, such was the intensity of that year and I'm sure this feeling might have grown had we not been successful at the fourth attempt, but who knows?

I'm glad we did do the fourth cycle of course. There were times we had thought about not doing so, especially as I wasn't in a positive place mentally, as I had been previously. Thank goodness we did! Some people have asked if I think the change in my mentality and approach made the difference, but I can't answer that question. Maybe? Maybe with the pressure off, it altered my body's make-up, but I'll never know and I would never suggest this was the reason to anyone. I'm just glad that we did take the plunge and though today it's hard work beyond my wildest dreams, I'm also glad we insisted on putting two embryos back too.

I know that the only time I felt relatively content was when we were in the midst of a treatment cycle and few people understood that this was the only tonic to my torment during those 13 months. Other distractions did nothing but frustrate me from what I wanted to focus on and what those around me tried to distract me with. I should have perhaps realised more, that other people didn't understand that. I got frustrated with them that they wanted to distract me, but how could they have understood how I felt? In my head I know now that I was unfairly cross at them, but it's easier to see that now, when I'm outside the intensity of the situation.

I can also now appreciate how difficult it really is seeing someone struggle with infertility, especially following a negative test, a period arriving, a failed cycle or indeed miscarriage or loss. There are no words to comfort, I know that first hand, and knowing that having someone there for you is sometimes all you need, still doesn't make it any easier when I'm on the other side, trying to work out how best to help and support someone going through it.

Looking back, I really feel for those who were around me in the darker days, it must have been extremely hard for them too. I can really see that the treatment affected many people around me more than I realised and at the time, cared. Yet I do care now, I feel almost guilty at the testing times I put friends, family and work colleagues through in my single-minded quest to get pregnant. I was selfish at times, I was hard to be around and undoubtedly there were occasions when those close to us were hurting too and didn't know how to console us. You can't have regrets, but it is only now when I look back that I realise how much we put other people through it too. I did everything I could, with family, amongst friends and at work, to be the very best I could be under the circumstances to be who, and what, they needed me to be. I'll never know if it was enough and I can't change those times, but I can appreciate now that life was far from normal for many people that were close to me during those challenging months.

As with many challenges life throws at you, you can't possibly fully understand until you are thrust in the situation yourself. People will always say or do the wrong thing because they are simply without the insight to know the correct thing to say or do – if that indeed exists. This was no different to any situation in life.

I know now that when people said "just remember, you have Zac" they were only trying to get me to focus on a positive. Such was my pain at the time, I could only feel anger and frustration, but that's perhaps more at their ignorance of the pain their words would cause, rather than at them as a person.

Zac is, as I knew he always would be, an amazing big brother. Xavi looks up to him in every way, he just wants to be like him copying his every move and wearing his clothes and football boots. Anya adores him, mothers him but also loves to play fight and tackle her brothers. It really is a noisy, hectic fun filled house that, in all honesty, drives me insane sometimes. Then I stand back, as I often do, listen to their chatter together, their laughter, their teasing and think yes, this was all that I dreamed of and so much more. Sometimes I look at Zac and the life he now has and wonder if he remembers what it was like before he had his brother and sister, that weirdly he predicted and asked for! I often wonder if he feels we did the right thing, if we made the right decision. What I do know is that he loves them as I knew he would and I am thankful daily for the three healthy kids that fill my life.

The right to have a second child should not be down to money, to whether you can afford to pay for the treatment. In the US, whether you can proceed with IVF depends on whether your insurance company covers fertility treatment and sadly many are surprised to learn it doesn't. In the UK, for those who are trying for a first child, where you live, currently determines how many IVF attempts you get for free on the NHS with differing health authorities offering different numbers with many reducing the number of cycles they are willing to cover. However, whether you had treatment the first time or not, if you already have had a child, you are not entitled to any free IVF treatment if you are struggling to conceive a second. We spent the best part of £20,000 in total to conceive our children, not a penny of which I regret, but it was a lot of money to find that other families simply do not have to.

We were lucky in that respect, we did have the money, but it breaks my heart to hear of those couples that aren't fortunate enough to have the money to try again, or indeed try at all, but whose instinct is no doubt still as strong as mine was. The World Health Organisation defines fertility as a "disease of the reproductive system" and yet treatment is not as readily available as it is for other diseases. And, where you haven't previously used NHS resources for a previous child, yet your reproductive system for some reason isn't working for a second child, this currently determines that you are not entitled to any free treatment? It doesn't make sense to me and I'm glad that Fertility Network UK is working hard to right what I believe is a wrong.

There are some people who will forever be in my heart and who I will always think about as my children grow up. The IVF team at Hull were an outstanding group of people who were highly skilled in their field, but were also exceptional at dealing with our needs as a couple. They knew when to focus, to be professional but they also knew when to laugh, to make me laugh and to make the whole process as easy as possible. Undoubtedly there are times when their job is extremely difficult, sad and frustrating and I regret those times for them when I know they want a positive outcome for every client. We share updates about the children with them, as well as the NICU team, and I hope our regular visits go some way to bring a smile as they see them all grow and make them realise how valued they really are.

Who knows why some couples get pregnant easily, some find it difficult and some just don't ever at all. There were no answers why we failed to conceive naturally or three times with IVF and that was always hard to accept. Yet perhaps what was harder was the fact that in the end, despite throwing everything and the kitchen sink at it, our success was possibly down to luck and fate. The fact that there isn't any pearl of wisdom that I can pass on to those about to start IVF that will really make any difference is extremely frustrating.

It would be easy to close this chapter of our lives, watch our children grow up and forget about a period that was painful and has now passed. Does it matter how our children came to be? Does any of it matter now that they are here, that our dream came true?

I felt guilty at my innermost thoughts and desires, I felt worthless that I couldn't do something for my son and I felt alone; the knowledge that I wasn't alone and that there are still couples struggling mean it does matter. It matters a lot.

Secondary Infertility matters because far too many couples are struggling with it. If the journey to having my children results in a legacy of helping just one of those couples, then, as painful as it was, it was indeed worth it and I am super proud of my family for inspiring us.

You are not alone. You should not feel guilty. It is OK to want another child.

Secondary Infertility Matters.

Acknowledgements

This book is about my story, my experience and my views but it is also largely a story I shared with my best friend, husband and wonderful father to my children, Jason. The man in the relationship is so often over looked, but this was his pain too. There were situations he found himself in where the reminder that we were struggling to conceive again was really painful. Whilst he didn't feel it as acutely or went through the treatment as I did, he did have to watch someone he loved go through it all and that must have been awful. Without him nothing would be possible. Jason is my rock, my grounding, my back up and the one who had to look at the side of my head for months whilst I tapped away on the laptop. I first remember thinking more seriously about Jason and our relationship when it dawned on me that he would make a great Dad to my kids, which was exceptionally important to me when considering a future husband. I chose well. He is an awesome Daddy, the best and I should remember to thank him more often for the 50% he put into our three wonderful, beautiful, amazing children. His support was immeasurable in writing this book and continues to be as I drive on my mission to raise the profile of Secondary Infertility.

It has been so strange talking about Zac whilst writing the book, blogging and being interviewed by the media when he has so little understanding about what it's all about. The little boy I mention is now growing up so fast into a mature young man and he is of course a wonderful big brother. My hope is that he will always have a close relationship with Anya and Xavi and that when he is old enough to understand, he will also realise how exceptionally blessed we all are to have each other. If he should ever question whether he was enough for us, I will easily respond that if he hadn't been so wonderful I would never have wanted another baby. May life bless your life Zac, as you have blessed mine.

Clearly I should acknowledge Anya & Xavier. Their arrival was the end of this story yet the start of a whole new life I began to think we would never have. Will they ever comprehend just how much we wanted them in our lives? What I want them to know more than anything when they are old enough to read this, is that it was worth it, every single bit of it was worth it and I'd have done more to be blessed with them. They are my dreams come true and I tell them every night as I tuck them in.

And how do you acknowledge the team who helped you achieve your family enough? Every single member of the Hull IVF Unit at Hull Royal Infirmary was exceptional in their professional expertise and wonderful care. Together we did it! I am super proud of the team and all they achieve week in, week out to help families achieve their dreams and especially for how they help those who are devastated by loss or failure. A special mention to Professor Killick, who has sadly since retired, who kept our chins up with his good humour and antics on each visit and to Denise Holland who has since been promoted to Director of the unit and Consultant Nurse and very deservedly so.

As I look back on our story whilst preparing the book, it is easy to see just how hard it must have been for those around me to know how best to support us. Liaising with couples still struggling with Secondary Infertility as I do now, I know at first hand how difficult it can be finding the right words. Sometimes there just aren't any. I'd like to thank my Mum, Andrew and Kate for their unfailing support when we needed it most.

If sisters were flowers, I'd pick Jo. For as long as I can remember she's been the big sister I never had and throughout this journey she was overwhelmingly generous with her love, advice and support. Sharing her own experiences with me and helping guide me through the minefield of fertility treatments was invaluable and I can only try to acknowledge what it meant to me by passing on this level of support through my website, blogs and monthly eshots to others.

I've also found that sometimes it's not the length of time you have known someone that makes you appreciate them but the impact they have on your life in the short time you have known them. Emma B, Karli and Sally M have been huge sources of energy and encouragement for me. Liking and sharing every post, high fiving every tiny step forward and always believing in me has massively helped give me the confidence to drive on.

We can laugh at some of the crazy antics my treatment got us into now, but on reflection, at the time, it must have been exceptionally tough on my business partners Emma and Dom. They saw it all at first hand and put up with a lot. From soothing me on the boardroom floor and holding me when I cried so many times, to printing out my precious babies names in a frame, they were immensely supportive.

To all the members of my team at work who tip toed round me, didn't ask questions when I looked dreadful and who put up with all the crazy antics, you clearly deserve a pay rise for what you tolerated so wonderfully. (I can say that now I don't own the business and most of you have moved on!)

We had friends who encouraged us, helped us out with Zac, picked me up and made me laugh when my heart was broken. Some have drifted away, some friendships remain stronger than ever, but none of what you did for us during those tough few years has been forgotten.

Big thanks to Jo Mac for proof reading every single one of the 102,000 words and for being considerate enough to apologise for each typo she found! Your care and attention to the detail was immense and your initial feedback gave me such a fabulous confidence boost.

Many thanks to Susan Seenan for kindly writing such an honest and inspiring foreword. I am honoured.

I'd like to mention Tone Jarvis-Mack, Publisher for Fertility Road magazine who was so willing to give me a shot in writing articles for his magazine that enabled me to reach out quickly and gave me the confidence to keep writing.

Duncan and Clare at YPS who showed me the way to publish my story and guided me through every stage. It's been an exciting time. Here's to the next one!

To all the girls who subscribe to my monthly support newsletter and who are members of my closed Facebook Group. This is your story too and I hope that in writing this book I can help reduce the stigma and misunderstanding of Secondary Infertility to relieve a little of the guilt I know you feel. Without hope we have nothing and I wish each and every one of you peace of mind and a full heart whatever your outcome.

To anyone still struggling with Secondary Infertility, hopefully this book has or will resonate with you and the message is clear for you. You are not alone, you should not feel guilty and there really are people who 'get you'. May you find the support and information you need.

And finally thank you to the publisher who turned me down and said "There isn't a market for this book." You lit a touch paper in me I never knew existed and prompted me to prove you wrong. There is unfortunately a huge market of couples across the world that will sadly appreciate, buy and benefit from this book and it is my intention to reach them. They may not know it yet, they may be unaware of the name of their condition, but without your rejection it would never have been my mission to tell them.